100 IDEAS FOR A CREATIVE APPROACH TO ACTIVITIES IN DEMENTIA CARE

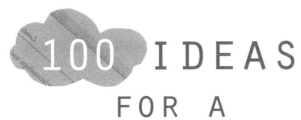

· · · · · · · · · · · · · · · · · ·

Written, designed and illustrated by

Sarah Zoutewelle-Morris

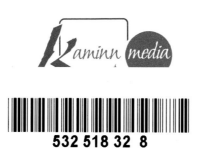

Kaminn Media
272 Bath Street
Glasgow G2 4JR
Scotland
kaminnmedia.com

2nd edition published by Kaminn Media in 2020

Previously published by Hawker Publications under the title
    *Chocolate Rain: 101 Ideas for a Creative Approach
    to Activities in Dementia Care*

British Library Cataloguing in Publication Data:
A CIP record for this book is available from the British Library

ISBN 978-1-912698-96-7 (print)
ISBN 978-1-912698-97-4 (ebook)

Illustrated and designed by Sarah Zoutewelle-Morris

Printed, bound and distributed by Ingram Spark

Neither the author nor publisher can accept responsibility for possible injury that could result from incorrect assessment or lack of supervision when carrying out the exercises in this book which involve sharp tools, or objects which could be swallowed.

TABLE OF CONTENTS

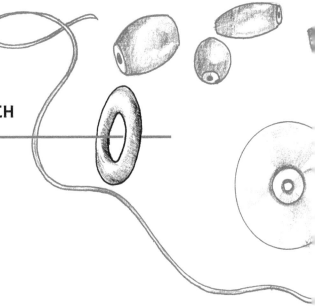

1 ELEMENTS OF A CREATIVE APPROACH

A CREATIVE APPROACH

ABOUT YOU

2 GETTING STARTED

3 CREATING YOUR OWN ACTIVITIES

HOME AND COMPANIONSHIP

WORKING, PLAYING, AND CREATING TOGETHER

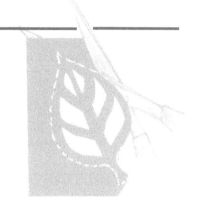

For my parents

*In many ways, the deepest revelation of the Alzheimer journey
is that it is a kind of passage from the mind into the heart.*
—Frena Gray Davidson

FOREWORD

I truly believe that at long last the time for the arts and dementia care has come. There are a number of signs, and this book is not the least of them.

What are its virtues? Well first of all it is user-friendly. It is not bulky to carry around. It is full of drawings that set you at your ease. It is written in a style that takes you into the writer's confidence. It is easy to absorb: the only thing that stands in your way is that it keeps asking you to try things out! That establishes it as a book to use and not to flip through or put on the shelf.

It is very basic – it takes nothing for granted. It is at the opposite pole from a text that is full of high-minded theories and generalisations: it says "This you can do!"

It pays particular attention to the needs of people with advanced dementia, especially those who rarely speak, and with whom it is difficult to make connections. Its definition of art is inclusive, and encompasses all sorts of activities that others might ignore as not being creative. This is a client-group that many commentators pass over because they do not know what to offer them. Sarah Zoutewelle-Morris certainly knows from long experience what can work.

In the poem 'The Bad Home' one lady said to me:

> Nothing to do, nothing to say.
> It's all blackness in front of me.
> Another thing, they just sit there
> And turn their thoughts inward.
> That's why we'll never get better.

Amongst other things, this is a cry for meaningful activity. With this book available there is no longer any excuse for tolerating this state of affairs.

—John Killick
author of *Poetry and Dementia*

Introduction

A small group of residents is sitting in the lounge of a care home, they are staring in front of them. The room is institutional: it is a large rectangle painted beige, and the walls are decorated with what looks like kindergarten art. A few old people are wandering aimlessly around the room. Everyone is locked in. The air is close and warm; there might be a TV on or a radio playing.
Staff occasionally come in to offer tea or coffee; sometimes a relative chats softly with one or two people. Maybe there is a scheduled group activity that day.

But generally and on a large scale, once clothed and fed, residents in various stages of dementia are left for long periods of time in impersonal environments with nothing to do and no one to talk to but the other residents.

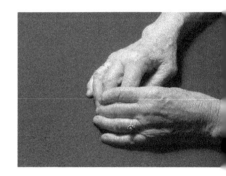

There are structural changes in the air, but before they are implemented on a large scale, existing conditions will continue. This book is about what we can do in the meantime to provide optimum attention to each person's social, emotional and spiritual needs.

As an artist doing project work in nursing homes and hospitals throughout Holland, I saw many old people with dementia in similar situations and their plight touched me deeply. I was convinced that with a more creative approach by everyone involved, these individuals could live meaningful lives, at home as well as in institutions.

Challenges

When I started working with people with dementia, here, in an agricultural area of northern Holland, I was convinced that my previous experience using art with diverse types of patients (including psychiatric geriatric) would be easily transferable. But the people I worked with in the new situation were neither conversant with the arts, nor did they understand my American accented Dutch. My carefully prepared activities were often sabotaged in the first few minutes when I took out art materials which the residents disdainfully rejected as being too 'childish' for adults.

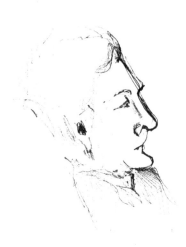

Denied my two most familiar means of communicating – talking and doing art, I was forced to find other ways to make contact. In the end it wasn't the cleverness of the project, the results, nor the materials that led to meaningful contact and successful activities. It was the degree to which on any given day I could be fully present and responsive to each person.
Where being an artist helped was in the generating of ideas, trusting those ideas to unfold in a process and following that process where it led.

For several years I worked weekly with people with this condition. I tried out dozens of ideas and I continually learned from the individuals themselves what would constitute a meaningful and pleasurable way to spend time together.

My intention in writing this book is to encourage you, the reader, to develop your own creative approach to communication and activity design for people with dementia.

Creativity 'disclaimer'

I should warn you that doing some of the exercises could bring unexpected positive changes not only to the life of the person with dementia but yours as well. You might experience insights that fundamentally change long held views, or hit upon a completely new form of self-expression that could release a chain-reaction of creativity in your life.

Suggestions for how to use this book

If someone were to hand you a list of 100 ideas on any subject, you'd have a good reference, but I doubt it would lead to you creating 100 ideas of your own.

Working interactively with this book should supply you with tools to enable you to keep coming up with new ideas. Indefinitely. This is because you will be developing your own creative abilities and once recognized, these are inexhaustible.

Though there are close to 100 illustrated activities with instructions included towards the end of the book (*100 activities handbook*), I've designed the sections to give you a chance to come up with your own ideas first. After completing some or all of the creative exercises in the section, *Creating your own activities*, you will end up with a group of ideas tailored to your situation.

Because the book devotes attention to exploring the creative process and how to come up with and implement your own ideas, you will be able to build on these inspirations as you go, developing not only new activities, but an entirely new approach to spending time with someone with dementia.

The book is divided into four main sections:
- **Section 1**
  an *introduction to the creative principles* upon which this book is based
- **Section 2**
  a selection of *tools and ideas* for getting started
- **Section 3**
  an *interactive section* with creative exercises to help you to get started writing your own ideas
- **Section 4**
  a collection of *100 ideas* for activities.

If you like to bounce around in a book rather than reading sequentially from cover to cover, it would still be a good idea to read the chapter, *Taking a step towards their world* (p16) because everything else is based on these ideas.

Then, you can dive right in to Section 3 (p66) and choose an activity category which seems easy and relevant to you, and do the creative exercises to get your inspiration primed.
You can use this book solo, in teams or as a group. Probably, the more people involved, the richer the variety of ideas you will have in the end.

Another option is to go to the *Mini-guide* section (p176) and look up a chapter which is relevant to you, for example, *Activities suited to men,* or *Activities for bedridden patients.* You can choose several ideas and read the section on how to implement them, or you could refer first to the *Activities List* (p180).

I've chosen a handbook format for easy reference and have left out long explanations about the disease. Several of the book recommendations in the bibliography contain more detailed information about dementia.

Too difficult?

At first glance, some of the art activities in the *100 activities handbook* section might seem too complex for someone with dementia. But as I will explain later in this book, activities have many purposes beside keeping someone occupied or achieving a goal.
The activity is a catalyst for establishing contact and keeping someone company in a mutually meaningful way.
Engaging in an activity in the person's presence is a way to start out from what 'can' be done. Only then does one make discoveries along the way that can be used to engage the person further.

Valuing the person with dementia

I don't see the person with dementia as an imperfect version of someone *without* dementia. She is a unique individual with a huge potential to surprise and teach me. Her brave attempts to communicate despite language failing her, her unexpected choice of words, and expressive behaviour all challenge me to meet her as a creative equal.

If you go from the assumption that things are possible, you'll bump into the solutions because you will either be looking for them or creating them.

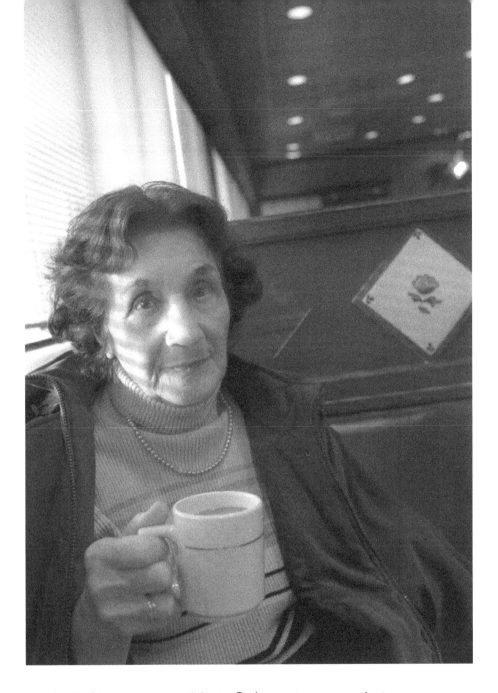

I am invited to use my creativity to find ways to communicate, validate and support that person where she is, as she is. During these encounters I learn to receive as well as give, to be as well as do, and witness as well as intervene. Like many others who work with people with this condition, each encounter has taught and enriched me.

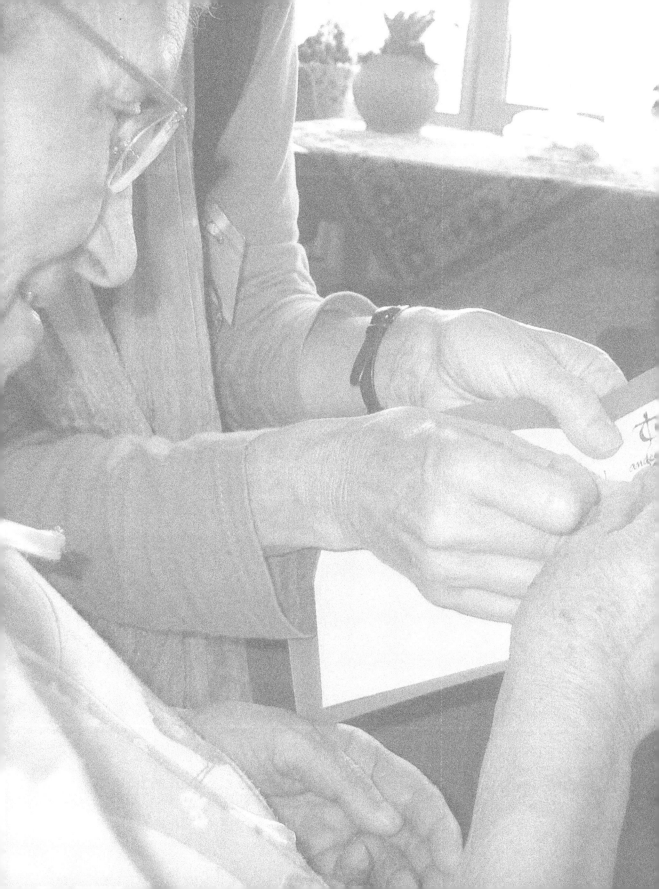

1

ELEMENTS OF
A CREATIVE
APPROACH

Taking a step towards their world

But I'm not creative

There are a lot of myths around creativity and talent, the dominant one being that only artists 'have it' and the 'rest of us' shouldn't even try. I've met many people who claim that they are 'not creative'. But in years of teaching various different visual disciplines I have never run across someone with the willingness to try who could not express themselves creatively.

Because our society is dominated by intellect, other less logical ways of perceiving are underdeveloped and are consequently undervalued. Among these are intuition, emotion, and imagination. All are central to art making. But they are also applicable to dementia care as we shall see later in this discussion.

Right and left brain

Our society is left brain based. The left half of the brain controls the rational, logical functions and the right brain is responsible for intuitive and 'imaginational' ways of perceiving.

You don't have to do art, sing or perform to be creative.

In the broadest sense, creativity starts with breaking away from 'the way things are always done' in order to discover or imagine fresh approaches.

This new way of seeing requires a shift in perception from logical reasoning to using the imagination. It doesn't mean that we abandon our intellects or logic, but that we consider right brained, more intuitive senses also to be valid. And we admit them into our world view.

Below are some left brained and right brained functions:

LEFT BRAIN HALF   RIGHT BRAIN HALF
Knowledge   Imagination
Rational thought   Feeling
Doing   Being
Science   Arts
Control   Letting go
Facts   Hunches
Planning   Letting unfold
Understanding   Intuiting

Ideally each person's world view would be in balance between intuitive as well as rational modes of perception.
But our education, especially Western medical training, is emphatically logic-based.
This kind of training creates literal-mindedness which in most cases insufficiently equips one to navigate the seemingly irrational terrain of dementia.

Unfamiliar terrain

The world of dementia at first may seem chaotic and threatening. It can be dominated by intense emotion. Symbolic gesture and language are used to communicate, objects are given new functions and can take on magical qualities, and language gains a new meaning or is lost altogether.

Caregivers who are comfortable operating from their creative as well as their professionally trained side are going to be more flexible, inventive and spontaneous when confronted with the unexpected twists and turns of the mind of someone with dementia.

Mr B in a care centre in Holland was becoming increasingly agitated because, he said, he needed to be at a business meeting in Cape Town, South Africa. A student nurse encountered him trying to get out of the ward and attempted to correct him by saying that he was in Holland, retired and no longer had to go to meetings. This only made him more angry.

In years of teaching different visual disciplines I have never run across someone with the willingness to try who could not express themselves creatively.

Characteristics of a creative approach

1 'Beginner's mind': maintain an open attitude free of judgment.

2 Be 100% available to the person and give them your full attention.

3 Approach the person from their potentials rather than their limitations.

4 Be process- rather than goal-oriented.

5 Authenticity rather than 'getting it right'.

6 Tolerance for uncertainty.

The caregiver who was finally able to soothe him was a male nurse who approached the man respectfully from within his situation. The nurse helped Mr B on with the coat kept on a rack in the hall for these kinds of situations, and walked with him, talking about his work and the meeting, until the urgency subsided.

I don't mean to imply that every situation is so easily resolved – sometimes nothing helps at all. Then all one can offer is kindness and understanding.

CREATIVE APPROACH

Based on a lifetime as a visual artist and several decades of art health care work, I've singled out some characteristics of a creative approach which I feel can be particularly relevant to care situations.

'Beginner's mind'

As an artist I need to approach each new subject I draw with an open mind. If I think I already know how something or somebody looks, I will be closed to the messages coming to me from the subject. Even if I have drawn an apple 100 times, I have never drawn *this* apple in this light, at this particular moment in time. Every single time I draw, I am invited to enter into a dialogue with what I am drawing and I learn from it.

Approaching someone with dementia with an open attitude invites us to enter this same kind of open dialogue. And it means emptying ourselves of preconceived notions about the person and the illness. It will be uncomfortable for professionals because it asks them to momentarily set some aspects of their training aside and approach the situation with the same curious, expectant attitude as a beginner.

Quality of Attention

Attention is perhaps the most denied gift of all –
to be completely available. In our heart of hearts each of us hopes
that there's someone to give us that.
Ferrucci P (2005)

The first thing an artist does when starting to draw, play music
or write a poem is to direct her undivided attention to the
subject. The rest of the creative act flows out of this state,
which is really a way of seeing things fresh every time.

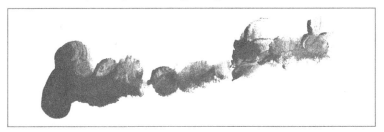

Mrs G came over and joined a group who were painting. She
dipped her finger in the paint began to smear it on the paper. I
handed her a brush and she dipped the 'wrong' end in some paint
and with deep concentration made some tight clots of paint in
an approximate line (see illustration). They weren't recognizable
forms but they had a dynamic pattern.
Eventually with her help I was able to decipher them as writing.
This was an epiphany for us both.
She had written her name and address, first with her fingers, then
with the 'pencil' end of the brush and lastly with the
end with the hairs.
(The words in pencil were added by her later as a clarification of
what she'd written with paint.)

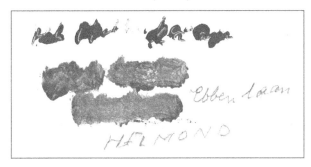

When you are giving someone your full attention you are free of judgment. You are simply present with them; there are no demands on them. The person will sense the spaciousness of this approach and will often open in new ways.

Accepting someone as they are without expecting them to be different leads to a special form of receptivity. This heightened alertness helps you pick up all kinds of cues from the person and situation that can be used as starting points for communication and activity. It lifts you out of the 'fixing' mentality and puts you an equal footing with the person so that together, you can discover what the best activity is.

Potentials: address the person, not the condition

Trusting the process is an open, highly sensitive response to the ever changing situation in front of you

A creative approach starts out from the potentials rather than the limitations of a situation.

Appraising someone in terms of their disabilities is literally debilitating.

Imaginative caregivers see past limiting beliefs about the people they care for. They take risks, try out new things, and begin with potentials instead of disabilities. They don't define the person by their illness and are constantly looking for ways of affirming the value of that individual.

Process oriented

Results are not the most important goal in activities for people with dementia. Focusing on results, in fact, can create stress as well as conditions where the person and caregiver can both 'fail'.

Each encounter and activity that I undertake with someone with dementia is open ended. I may have a particular direction I'd like to move in, but I don't hold to it rigidly.

If, during the process, something else starts to happen, I follow where it leads.

For example:

I gave Mr N a pencil and paper to write with. He ignored the paper and rolled his tie around the pencil then rolled it back down again, becoming fascinated with this movement. I got some wooden dowels for him and strips of cloth and rope; he wrapped several dowels in cloth and tied them. He 'worked' all morning.

Shaun McNiff (1998) repeatedly refers to the 'creative-intelligence' inherent in every situation. He describes it as a force both within and outside of the creator which 'knows' the appropriate path to take.

Trusting the process is an open, highly sensitive response to the ever changing situation in front of you.

Authenticity as opposed to getting it 'right'

Creativity is inherently messy, unpredictable, and not subject to control – not unlike dementia really.

When I teach drawing or calligraphy to adults, 'perfect' drawings are not the goal. I look instead for a lively personal line, and risk-taking, i.e. not falling back on a formula that has worked before.

Similarly, when doing an art activity with a person with dementia my focus is on gestures and spontaneous mark-making rather than only representational art. This creates a no-fail environment where people can start to loosen up and feel free to try new things.
Authentic expressions are rarely 'pretty' or pleasing in conventional ways, but they have a raw beauty all their own. Assessing artwork in this way requires a shift out of our normal modes of seeing, but it can be learned.

Maybe this appreciation for imperfection and authenticity also helps in accepting people with dementia exactly as they are. In this context, seemingly 'strange' behaviours are not seen as problems but accepted as raw material to create with.
(See Start where they are p104, and Activities based on gestures p166.)

Tolerance for uncertainty

Working continually with the creative process develops a tolerance for sustained uncertainty. I can never be sure when starting out where I will end up. Often in the middle of a creative process things break down into chaos before they regroup in a new configuration. It takes a good deal of trust and experience to navigate these chaotic periods and wait until they resolve themselves.

Encounters with people with dementia can take unexpected turns, throwing us into uncertainty. But with practice, one learns to move with the rhythm of an interaction whilst maintaining one's own stability. Or to withdraw if necessary.

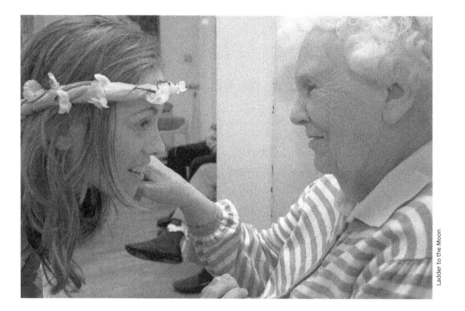

Ladder to the Moon

In a creative approach to communicating with people with dementia the primary goal is not to accomplish anything. The idea is to enter into a moment together and see what happens. I spend time with someone in a dynamic way: all my senses are alert to what the person may be trying to communicate and my capacities are sharpened in order to help them do that.

Creative stance

Here are some examples of creative attitudes at work, in an encounter with someone with dementia:

The creative worker

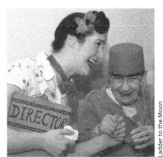

- Approaches the person openly, free of prejudice about what they supposedly can and can't do: files away other people's assumptions about limitations and relies on own sensibilities to assess the person's abilities

- Acknowledges and supports the person's potentials and existing abilities

- Keeps alert and focuses attention on the person, noting their present state of mind and the state of their surroundings

- Improvises with the situation at hand

- Takes risks and enters unknown territory by staying present and responding to bizarre or confusing behaviour in a calm, centred way

- Accepts 'nonsense' gestures, speech and sounds as valid efforts at communication and tries to respond to them

- Apologises for her own shortcomings if she fails to understand what they are trying to say

- Plays, explores, participates

- Relaxes role as caregiver/giver, is open to receiving

- Lets rational self take a back seat and trusts what intuition and senses are saying

- Accepts playing the fool and getting into absurd situations – lets sense of humour guide.

The **results**
this approach
encourages are:

- Increased trust

- Heart to heart contacts

- Prolonged moments of lucidity

- Calm rather than agitated behaviour

- Initiative taking by person with dementia

- Enhanced memory function

- Active participation

- Communication

- Increased frequency of physical contact

- Learning new skills

The person with dementia

Empowering the person with dementia

One of the aims of this book is to eradicate all possibility of 'excess disability' which is the worsening of someone's condition as a result of how they are treated or poor conditions in their care or environment.

The ideas for activities provide ways to be with someone in a respectful way on equal footing and to spend mutually enjoyable time doing meaningful activities suited to an adult.

Even though the word is still widely used, repeatedly referring to someone as 'demented' is negative because it defines them exclusively by their illness. On the other hand if you simply say, 'person with dementia', as you would refer to a 'person with cancer' or any other disease, you address the person first, and the illness second.

Empowering someone is different from helping them because it approaches them from their strengths and not their limitations. You approach them as an equal and explore together what the possibilities are.

People in nursing homes are surrounded with 'helpers' which automatically confines their own role to 'receivers of help'. One of the most empowering things you can do for someone in this position is to provide an opportunity for them to help you or to help themselves.

When language and function betray the sick, leaving them without the ability to say what they mean, the only thing left is action.

Acting out becomes a symbolic portrayal of their truth.

In years of [working with people with dementia] I have never come across a problem behaviour that did not arise from unmet needs or poor handling by carers.

—Frena Gray Davidson (1995)

24

All the activities in this book can be done in a way that people's strengths and potentials are emphasized. Their aim is not to 'keep someone busy' but to enrich and support the individual with dementia where they are, as they are.

Dementia is an extremely disempowering situation. For those still living at home, the activities are designed to bring stability and normality to a world that has been turned upside down with the loss of cognitive abilities.
And for people in an institutional setting, the activities are meant to give them a sense of home, genuine companionship and a sense of autonomy.

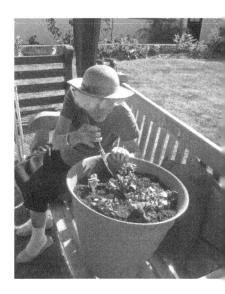

Many kinds of logic
Jitka Zgola tells a story, set in a psychiatric nursing home.

A man repeatedly tried to get into bed with a woman at a certain time of night. After careful analysis and talks with the man's family, it appeared that this was not a case of promiscuity, but of a simple mistake in logistics.

When the man got up at night to use the toilet, he then returned to what he thought was his own bed, which at home had been to the left of the bathroom, and in the nursing home, his room was to the right. The woman's bedroom was where he thought his room should be.
His logical reasoning was in perfect order, only the reality didn't fit it. Zgola (1999).

There are countless stories of this kind, where individuals are acting according to, for them, a perfectly sensible logic. But because of our prejudices about dementia and because we lack certain facts, we classify their behaviour as irrational or worse.

I am not claiming here that all behaviour of people with dementia can be interpreted this way, but there is certainly a long way to go before we have exhausted the possibilities of understanding what makes someone do or say a certain thing.

If you can imagine yourself as the person with dementia, how would you want to be approached? If someone related to you as a whole, reasonable person, you'd have the opportunity to express yourself in an unpressured way. On the other hand, if people would repeatedly treat you like a crazy person who utters only nonsense and does bizarre things, there is a good chance you might get frustrated and start displaying some 'problem behaviour'. I would!

That is why the main plea of this book is to learn to use and value our imaginations just as much as our intellects when interacting with individuals with this condition. By putting ourselves in their shoes and trying to intuit what it is they are trying to express, we are already showing respect for that person and giving them a chance to communicate to us.

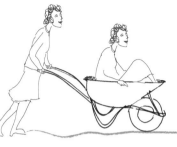

Bringing yourself along

'My mother is deaf and her vision is failing. She is bedridden and not very aware – she doesn't even seem to know who I am. Why should I keep coming to visit and what can I do when I'm there?'

It can be daunting to spend time with a person whose mental and physical capacities are deteriorating and who can no longer participate in 'normal' conversation or activity. But the real tragedy is when families give up at this stage and stop visiting.

In terms of communication, the advanced stages of dementia are extremely challenging for everyone involved. Yet, I feel that there is always a part of the person beyond the symptoms which can be addressed.
I've repeatedly seen individuals who were generally unresponsive, perk up when a loved one visited. And even when there is no visible outer change, how can anyone know conclusively that a caring presence does not bring comfort?

In a ward for advanced dementia patients there was a woman who had been bedridden for years:

Greta lay on her back in a row of beds, hour after hour, day after day looking up at the ceiling. Her only social contact was being bathed and dressed by her caregivers. She could not speak, though I found her very present when eye contact was made. It was hard to know how to engage her, or if she even desired this.
Every week, though, her sister would travel up by train for 3 hours each way to see her. She brought freshly squeezed fruit juices and flowers and would talk to her bedridden sister during her entire visit, bringing her up to date with family news.

It was a normal family visit and I saw how much good it did the patient and the sister.

Relations and friends are often the last links the person has left to her disintegrating familiar world and they have the important, and I think, precious role of holding that person's past in safekeeping for them.

Caregivers can also play an important part in supporting someone's identity. Through day to day contact a degree of familiarity is built up. As you become more comfortable with using your imagination during the tasks of daily care, your attention can make a positive difference in someone's life.

Words

Though talking is our natural way of communication, when words cease to make sense to the affected person, we simply need to find other ways to communicate. Whatever your relationship to the person with dementia, you have a lot more resources to draw on than you first may think.

Granted, most of the suggestions below use words, but in such a way that they demand no response. In this manner you create a gentle flow of comforting words and even if the person doesn't grasp the exact meaning, you are validating them by speaking to them and including them in a social interaction.

Here are some suggestions for spending time with someone with cognitive impairment:

Greet the person clearly, say who you are if necessary and say why you've come and perhaps mention what you intend to do. This may simply be, 'I've come to visit you and just sit here awhile today. Or maybe we could go for a walk, the weather is nice.'

If you are sitting in a room or lounge, check if they appear comfortable: in a subtle respectful way, see if their basic physical needs have been met such as going to the toilet. See if their clothes are comfortable, not too tight, or too warm.

Position yourself in such a way that both of you are comfortable and can see each other well. Is the person hard of hearing on one side? Take this into account when you sit down.

Are they in bed? Sit where they can see and hear you comfortably.

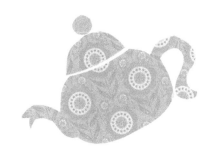

Starting out with a cup of tea is a nice ritual. It gives you something to do to bring you there fully, it is an act of welcome and friendship, and you don't have to think of things to say right away.

Practise just being there. Being there gives you a chance to feel what is needed today, for you, and for the person you are with. See the next chapter, *Being there.*

Ice breakers

A simple opening sentence like, 'How are you today?', includes the person immediately in a social interchange. Or you could try an observation, 'I've seen that dress before, it suits you well, I love the blues and purples together. Do you? Look, it is the same colour as these flowers on the table'.

Be alert to what is happening in the environment. Maybe it is someone's birthday and there is cake for everyone, or there might be some scheduled event at the home which you may want to attend or avoid.

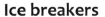

If there is a TV or radio on all the time the extra stimuli can short-circuit the person's ability to focus. It might be appropriate to take your friend, mother, the patient, out of the lounge to a quieter place. Or you could put on quiet classical music or nature sounds to bring some calm to the surroundings.

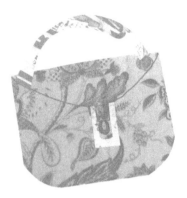

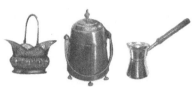

Show and tell

Bring along tangible things from your life to share, photos, plants, interesting objects from their life or yours. Bring something to do that can involve the other – even if it is only as a spectator sharing the interesting process of creating something. More on this in the chapter *Making things for/with*.

Second hand shops

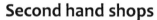

I was always on the lookout for interesting items for my group. Here are a few I picked up over the years:

- various relevant picture books, for example, *Oceangoing vessels* for ex-Captain R
- a full set of antique miniature copper utensils that were an endless source of stories and associations
- some wonderful old costume jewelry and scarves which were passed around among the women for months
- and finally, old wallets and purses. These last items were in big demand; people liked the responsibility of having a wallet or purse again. I helped them fill it with coins and important looking papers containing their address, name and other information they found pertinent.

Granted, these objects were sometimes left, forgotten or taken by other residents (often on the same day they were received), but that is simply part of the risk with dementia. The moment of giving was not lost, though. And even if they didn't remember the specifics, the people I worked with came to associate my arrival with discovery and fun.

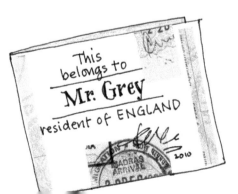

This belongs to **Mr. Grey** resident of ENGLAND

Exercises

1   List three interests of yours and a way you could share them with a resident/
patient. (Tip: bring in scented herbs or plants from your garden and let people
smell them, talk about associations with 'lavender' for example.)

2   Which of your family anecdotes might be relevant to the person you are
with? Include them as you tell them about it.

3   Is there a story or poem you could tell or read to someone? Even if 100% com-
prehension is not present, it can be comforting to be read to. Your facial expression and intonation can convey a lot about the meaning behind the words.

4   What is your most natural way of communicating? Try a new way
slightly outside your comfort zone, perhaps singing. (Tip: if talking is your
usual way, you could listen to music together or you could try being silent and
touching, if appropriate.)

5   Bring in an iPod or other music player and share some of your favourite music
with them. If you are young let them hear what your generation is listening to,
the least you can get is a laugh!

6   If you are familiar with the place the resident came from, they might like to
know about recent happenings or gossip. Support the story with photos or
other props.

7   Are you redecorating your home? Or are you involved in any other project that
provides a good 'before and after'? Bring in pictures of the process.

8   New babies are great subject matter for most people. Pictures, the child herself,
or videos are fun.

9   I once spent a whole afternoon showing three ladies the wonders of my
new cell phone. For them it was magical: they had heard about my husband, now
they could each speak to him. Do you have a similar gadget to wow people with?

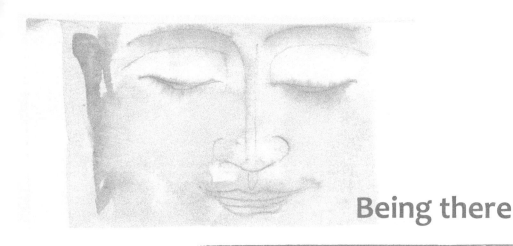

Being there

One day, during my first month working at the home, I stood in the middle of a ward at a complete loss for what to do next. Around me, against the walls, were seven beds, each containing a person in the last stages of dementia and their lives. I'd already tried out different ways to contact these individuals, sometimes with success; but on that day I was fresh out of ideas.

What I really wanted to do was give up and go home, and leave this depressing room full of dying, disoriented people.
The exact moment that I fully accepted this feeling and admitted defeat, one of the residents from another wing wandered in, and gave me a gentle comforting pat on the back. This woman was usually withdrawn and known for her aggressive flare-ups, so her empathy took me completely by surprise.
She actually stood in front of me looking at me until she saw that I felt better, then she said, 'Good', turned around and left.

If I hadn't reached that point of giving up, I doubt I would have been open enough to receive that unexpected gift from Mrs W. That day my inspiration didn't return, so I just sat quietly with one woman by her bed. And that was fine.

Being there is a lost art
We feel so compelled, especially in the role of caregiver, to always 'Do Something'. We have lost the capacity to sit still and be comfortable with just doing nothing, and even more importantly, to see that as a valid part of our work.
There are ways to quietly spend time with someone that can be deeply nourishing for both parties.

One of the first things 'just being there' can accomplish is to allow the person with dementia time to initiate something. Often people with dementia respond to stimuli in a delayed fashion. Learning to quietly wait and see if more words or gestures are coming helps the person to relax and perhaps seek contact with you.

Silence
Often we plan so much because we are uncomfortable with inactivity and the accompanying silence.

Dissatisfied with the constant bombardment of media, emails, radios, videos, TV, billboards, and small talk, increasingly more people are paying good money to go on silent retreats. The first days in the retreat centre or monastery are, for most, very uncomfortable. But gradually, as the mind is released from constant chatter it eventually settles, and many people experience profound peace.

Start with the situation in front of you
Begin where they are. Before you can 'DO' something with someone you need to have your antennae out to assess the situation you are entering.

When you come into the room and greet your friend or loved one with dementia, just stop for a moment. Sit down, take in the room, the person, the atmosphere. Feel what is happening in the whole facility, maybe people are running to and fro, or there is tension, or it is unusually quiet. Is there an emotional cloud hanging when someone has just died? Are there unspoken issues that may need to be addressed?

Pay attention to your breathing, quiet your thoughts, and feel your body. Become aware of the breathing of the person you are visiting.

Is this a time of day when the person is alert, or do they need to rest?

Silence, they say cannot be written.
Bullfrog:

"Garronk"

Scale the activity accordingly. If they are present but not too sharp, taking a walk or listening to music might be best. Silence can have different qualities; and indeed, just sitting with someone without 'doing' can be awkward.

But practice in accepting the discomfort of silence will make a real difference in the quality of the time spent with someone. It enables one, for instance, to go for a walk without constantly making small talk. In general your tempo and demeanour will become gentler, slower, more responsive. The majority of communication happens non verbally, and it is likely that the mood of whomever you are with will adjust to the level of calm you are projecting.

Emptiness is the state from which creativity emerges. 'Being there' entails trusting that you will know what to do next even if you don't know it now.

Often, all that the person with dementia has is the present moment, the Now. We, on the other hand, tend to live in our minds in either past events or future conjecture.
When we join the person with dementia here and Now, we are given a gift. Life can open out in an unexpected way when we open to the richness of just one moment at a time.

According to some spiritual teachers, life is an eternity of such Now moments. Tolle E (1999) *The Power of Now*.

Exercises

1   Right now, stop what you are doing and just sit. Pay attention to your breathing, feel your body on the chair, notice your thoughts. Sit quietly and do nothing. A minute or two now is fine, try building up to five minutes of inaction. If this brings you into a state of peace try to return to it at other times in the day.

2   Practise a day of 'reading deprivation' to get an idea of how we constantly fill up our time with word-related activities. In *The Artist's Way*, by Julia Cameron (1994), one of the tasks to developing one's creativity is a whole week of reading deprivation; it is a powerful exercise which reveals how opportunities for creative activity and reflection can be displaced by the habit of going to the computer, TV, magazine or a book just to waste time.

3   Observe the other person's breathing and harmonise your breathing with theirs. Do this for as long as it feels comfortable.

4   Bring along some handwork or sewing to do while you are sitting with the person. Include them in the process by showing and telling what you are doing. But if they are in a restful mood, don't ask them to participate.

5   What else could you bring to do which would leave your attention mostly free to be present with them?

Reflection

If you are past a certain age you may experience, as I have, short memory lapses. These are normal, but provide brief glimpses into what might be like to have dementia.

Several years ago, on a routine trip to take money out of the bank wall dispenser, I forgot my pin code of ten years. I tried various combinations until the machine threatened to block my card, but no amount of willing would bring back the sequence of four numbers. The complete though temporary loss of a piece of automatic information was a shock to me.

This chapter is important to communication and activity design because it will give you insights into what it must be like to gradually lose your hold on reality. These insights can heighten your sensitivity and alertness as a caregiver or companion for someone who must live every day in a world of broken connections.

Following are some exercises to help you remember or imagine similar moments. If you take the time to do this, your under-standing of your loved one or patient/resident will increase and so will your capacity to support them.
The exercises are most effective if done with another person or completed in writing.

As we discover the person who has dementia we also discover something of ourselves.
For what we ultimately have to offer is not technical expertise but ordinary faculties raised to a higher level; our power to feel, to give, to stand in the shoes of another, through the use of our imagination.
—Tom Kitwood (1993)

Exercises

Please take a moment to reflect on the following:

1   Remember a time when you forgot:
     a. an appointment
     b. someone's name
     c. where you put your keys or glasses

2   Did you ever mistake a common object for something else? For example, you think you see a snake in the woods, but it turns out to be a rope.

3   Have you ever lost your way on a once familiar street, or turned a corner and suddenly lost your bearings?

4   How does it feel when you can't remember a certain word?
     Do the exercise below quickly without thinking too much, as if you were in a conversation and had to come up with the word on the spot:
     a. Find a substitute word or phrase for the following words instantly. (Example: *rain* – 'the drops that come out of a cloud') *car, clock, thimble, cat, bowl*

5   Have you ever woken up in an unfamiliar room and not known for a moment where you are? Go back to that feeling and describe it.

6   Friends are discussing an event in which you also took part. You recognize the story, but remember some elements completely differently from their version. Both parties are sure of their version. How does this feel?

7   Has anyone ever told you that you didn't do something you were sure you had done? What is the feeling?

8   What did you eat for dinner a week ago?

...OUT AND PASTING ...IMAGES, etc

INTO YOUR NOTEBOOK.

...ook will eventually fill up
...your unique impressions.
...g through it you will see
...sly vague ideas in a
...le form which can be
...d, arranged, & changed.

THIS M...
BECOMES...
SOURCE F...
NEW IDEAS...
WHICH CAN...
SPILL OVER I...
OTHER AREAS
OF YOUR LIFE

* some of the quot...
& sketches in thi...
from my ide...

*

2

GETTING STARTED

Purpose and characteristics of activities

The question that drives my professional practice will always be: what can I do to improve the quality of life for someone with dementia. Biernacki C (2009)

Despite the introduction of more homelike environments and person-centred care for people with dementia, once clothed and fed, residents in countless care centres are still left for long periods of time with nothing to do.

One of the ironies of our times is that our society removes people from everything that nourishes them – their homes, neighborhoods, and roles in the family, confines them to institutions, then has to contrive 'activities' to fill up all that emptiness.

It will be a long time before the systems change significantly enough to provide optimum attention to each person's social, emotional and spiritual needs. I hope this book will provide inspiration for what we can do in the meantime.

In my work as an artist in healthcare, I go around hospitals and nursing homes carrying a box filled with craft supplies for perhaps ten different kinds of activities. While it is important to fit the activity to each person I encounter (bedridden, active, child, or adult etc.), I have discovered that the essential factor is not what I do, but the quality of contact that is established between myself and the patient. It is from this relationship that true care, communication, and meaningful activity flow. One individual's positive intent can make an enormous difference in the life of someone with dementia.

Purposes of an activity

A creative approach to activities calls into question many of our assumptions about what constitutes a good activity, the primary one being that an activity's main purpose is to 'keep someone busy'.

I have come to understand that activities can have multiple purposes.

For example an activity can be a way to:
- establish contact and give attention
- spend time with someone enjoyably
- strengthen and support someone's identity
- stimulate someone to use the abilities they have and to learn new ones
- create a sense of home and normality.

CHARACTERISTICS OF A GOOD ACTIVITY

Just about anything can be an activity: tearing paper, feeling textures, moving something from one location to the other, arranging objects, drinking tea together, walking somewhere, etc. I've found that one-to-one, simple activities work well. The activity needs to be no-fail, pleasurable for both parties, suited to the person's age, status and gender, and should be perceived by them to be meaningful or useful.

For hesitant individuals, I tend to start with an activity that is engaging enough to stimulate them but doesn't require active participation right away. I begin the process then invite them to join in or help me as I work.

One to one

There is quite a bit of material available on the benefits of group activities in care centres. I prefer working one to one, especially on art/craft projects because I can give concentrated personal attention to help the person fulfill the task.

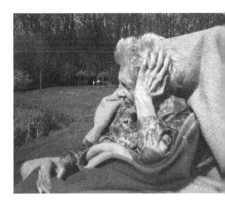

Grass

A young fella carried me
in here, it were a long way
and a long time ago.
I were lying on grass...

I don't want to stay, no
there's nothing for me
they're all very kind
but I don't want to be

inside anywhere at all
it's much too hot and bright
it just don't feel right
I've not been used

I need the fresh air
I keep calling out:
nurse, nurse, carry me
outside to where

I were lying on grass...

—as told to and recorded by
John Killick from
You are words,
Dementia Poems, (1999)

Simple

Activities don't have to be elaborate or expensive to succeed. One of the simplest activities I've done was to fill a dishpan with warm sudsy water.
I brought it around to four different women who each did something different with it.

The first woman was a conscientious homemaker and we washed and dried dishes. The second resident simply liked the feel of the warm soapy water, and she made happy sounds as she played with my hands underwater. One woman wanted to wash her doll's clothes, and her reading glasses. And the fourth played with the suds and gave me a hand massage afterwards.

Pleasurable for both parties

Try to choose something that you are interested in – games, crafts, grooming, reading out loud. What feels natural to do in your relationship with the individual? If the person's condition means that there is not much common ground to start from, use your creativity to help you adapt to the new situation.
For example: Your aunt always played cards, but no longer understands the rules of the games. Develop a new game such as *Memory* using a normal deck. Or build or make things with the cards.

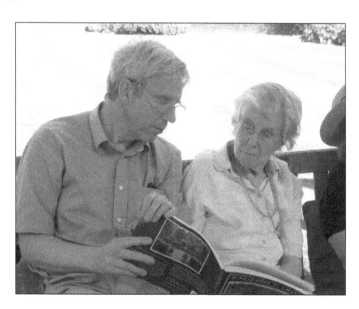

Memory variation: If the person can't remember the position of the card she just turned over, instead of returning the card to its face-down position, you can leave the card exposed until she finds the match. Reducing the deck by half can facilitate this game. Please also see the *Games & play* (p84) and *Activity grading* (p48).

Suited to the person's status, age and gender

Because their lack of cognitive skills may put them back at the basics of language, communication and other abilities, some people think of people with dementia as children. But they are emphatically not children; they are legitimate adults with a lifetime of experience behind them.

I remember when my grandmother, a highly cultured Parisian who also composed music and played the piano was in a nursing home. We were at a birthday party with silly hats, treats, and music: all of this was more suited to a group of five year olds than the varied adult population present. Grandmère hadn't been communicating much, but at one moment her eyes met mine and exchanged a look with me that said it all – ie what a total insult to her intelligence and dignity this activity was.

Activities can be based on former professions, though one sometimes has to tread carefully if there is frustration associated with lost skills or other aspects of former work.
The office folder is one example of an activity designed for former office managers or others who enjoy arranging papers and handling office supplies (p126).

Mrs van D was a natural organizer and always tried to appropriate the folder and papers I had with me.
So I made a folder for her, containing many papers and materials she could discover, read, and arrange. It included gift cards, name tags, paper clips, a page of paint colour samples, an old letter from my bank, and scraps of my old artwork.

Characteristics of a good activity

1 One to one
2 Simple
3 Mutually pleasurable
4 Suited to the person's status, age and gender
5 Meaningful/useful
6 No-fail

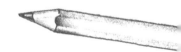

A ps to this story which reveals the sometimes unfathomable world of dementia is that after I'd left it for her and sneaked a satisfied peek at her using it, I came in at the end of the day to find it lying on the table. When I opened it, I discovered she had used it to conceal something of her own; perfectly centred on the right hand side of the folder, and only slightly squashed, was a juicy slice of pear.

Meaningful or useful

On occasion, when I've offered an activity like making a collage, some people in my group weren't convinced that they were doing something functional. When the process of 'just making something' is not enough, add a theme or goal:

No-fail means that every word, every gesture, every attempt is valued, counted and appreciated.

- Collage on a theme like 'Summer', or 'Breakfast'
- Greeting cards: make one for a particular season or person
- Making decorations, show the person where they will be hung up or placed
- Present finished poems in a simple book form or mount them on coloured paper and hang them up (p132,133)
- If you've just organized a yarn drawer, go to the activity room together where the finished result can be admired. Refer to it later; even if the person doesn't remember the specifics they will be able to re-experience the sense of accomplishment.

I discourage doing pointless tasks. I heard of one home where socks were brought in to be paired, that's fine but the pairs were taken away and brought back again loose 15 minutes later – to be done again!

No-Fail

No-fail doesn't mean dully unimaginative like the socks above. It means open-ended tasks without a 'right' or 'wrong' solution. Every word, every gesture, every attempt is valued, counted and appreciated.

When the goals are to give someone attention, support them where they are, and spend quality time together, no failure is possible.

We were gathered round a table making tissue paper collages. A resident from another wing wandered in and began spiriting away large strips of coloured paper. He would come back in, sidle up to the table and take another one. I began leaving him torn, folded, crumpled and other interestingly altered bits of paper which he carried away one by one all afternoon.

Creative approach

A creative attitude starts out with a sincere and unshakable belief in the potentials of anyone, regardless of their cognitive capacities, to express themselves.
And this approach is at the heart of successful interaction and pleasurable activities.

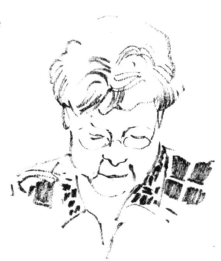

Through my work in hospitals and nursing homes over the years, I've found that the starting points of every creative encounter, whether an art activity or washing someone, are: respect for the person, support for their autonomy, and celebrating that person as they are.

If this attitude is not at the core of an encounter none of the activities I've described here will go beyond superficially 'keeping someone busy'.

Mind to heart

It has been said that dementia is a journey from the mind to the heart, and this is not just addressed to the person with dementia.
In embarking on the following exercises, I think you will discover that it isn't your expertise as much as your humanity and imagination that will ease the difficulties of this complex illness.
I hope that this book brings you and your loved one or patients many hours spent together in mutually enjoyable activity.

Staying involved

How do you keep your interest level up during activities that
may seem meaningless or childish?

First it is important to reflect again on the goals for doing activities with persons with dementia. As opposed to the usual pur-
poseful or 'productive' ways of accomplishing things, we are
aiming first of all to create a sense of normality and security.

Though I discourage comparisons between people with dementia and children, in this case the quality of attention needed to
be with a cognitively impaired person is comparable to a mother's in the early years of raising her child. The difference is that
children are an obvious investment in the future, while people
with dementia are more often written off as nothing more than
ageing bodies to be maintained. But we need to challenge the
prevailing opinion and assert that people with dementia can be
stimulated to preserve their abilities as well as learn new ones.

I have experienced that spending quality time can have deep
and lasting therapeutic effects on people with this condition.
Please see the sidebar on page 23 for some of these benefits.

★ Rewards

As for you, the caregiver, the rewards of learning to act from a
state of calm, patient, alert attention are subtle but many.
For example:
- Learning to 'just be' brings inner peace and can
  lower stress.

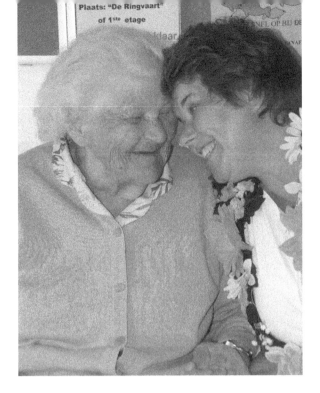

- Activities approached this way create an opportunity for the individual to give to you, and for you to receive from them.

- The time spent changes from boredom and obligation to genuinely being engaged. You leave refreshed rather than drained.

- You gain skills in working with people with a cognitive impairment which can be applied in other situations.

- And finally, developing your own creative abilities contributes to personal growth and enrichment and can be applied to other aspects of your life.

So, the next time you are bored with just sitting with someone, you could try seeing it as a meditative exercise. Let all your scattered thoughts settle, accept the moment and the situation and agree to be fully present. Feel open to receiving inspiration from wherever it comes.

Activity grading

Activity grading is scaling the activity to fit it to an individual's current level of ability. This is done in order to enable each person to participate in and enjoy an activity whatever their level of ability. (There are suggestions for activity grading throughout this book.)

I remember the first time, laden with all kinds of craft materials, I entered a family room in a unit for people with advanced dementia; I received kind but sceptical looks from the nursing staff. And indeed, at first I found that making even a simple paper flower was beyond the scope of many residents.

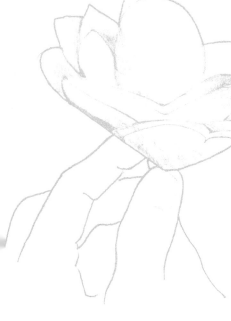

However, as I came back with my materials week after week, people got used to me and when encouraged, began to try things. And even though only a small percentage of the group could actually complete a project, everyone could be drawn in at some level and made to feel that they contributed something.

There is a role for everyone
The following list is adapted from *Care that works* by Jitka Zgola (1999).
Baking cookies is usually a group activity done in the family room, and there is a range of participation available for each individual. The list below begins with the most complex tasks, organising and planning, and modifies the task step by step as cognitive abilities diminish. It is good to keep in mind that a person's capacities can vary; someone who can't actively participate today may well be able to do so tomorrow.

Baking cookies

Someone with intact cognitive abilities (usually in an early phase of the condition) can take on an organising and implementing role. She or he can decide on the kind of cookies, choose a recipe, plan, shop, and/or bake.

Independent organiser-doer

Individuals who are not able to take the initiative or plan can, once the ingredients have been prepared for them, take over and make the cookies.

Independent doer

A person who cannot complete the task of making the cookies on their own can do the whole task with supervision/help.

Doer with supervision

If the person can't remember in sequence enough to complete a whole task with supervision, they can do a specific step like: measuring, mixing, pouring, or forming the cookies, depending on ability and affinity for the task.

Doer of a specific task

If doing a specific task alone is too hard, the individual can repeat one small step such as stirring, with help or supervision.

Doer of a modified task

If repeating a task with help isn't working well, they can listen for the oven timer to go off, clean up pieces of dough, put utensils back, and help washing up.

Observer-monitor

Persons who don't want to or cannot participate in the above-mentioned ways, can be consulted about their own experience or expertise, or memories (even if it has nothing to do with baking).

Observer-advisor

There will always be one or more individuals who want to sit quietly and watch; they can be the cookie taster.

Observer-critic

And people who are not willing or able to participate in any of these ways can still watch or listen whilst being made to feel part of the occasion. They may be given a piece of dough to handle or taste, their opinion may be asked, or they may simply be informed of the proceedings by you saying, 'OK, Mrs B watch, I'm going to add the chocolate chips now'.

Observer

Exercises

Break down one of the following activities into the categories below:

- *Making a simple collage,*
- *Cleaning out and organising a sewing box*
- *Cleaning out and organising a tool box.*

CATEGORIES

Independent organizer-doer

Independent doer

Doer with supervision

Doer of a specific task

Doer of a modified task

Observer-monitor

Observer-advisor

Observer-critic

Observer

Creative thinking
how to generate ideas

In the introduction to this book I spoke about elements of a creative approach, including keeping an open attitude and focusing on the process rather than the end result.

The next section of activity categories invites you to use this creative approach to think up activities tailor made for your particular situation.

All the categories begin with an introductory text followed by an exercise section.

For example, the category, *Making something for/with* introduces ideas for applying visual art/craft as a way to spend meaningful time with someone. In the exercise section for this category you are invited to think of topics for: collage themes, activities based on former hobbies of a resident, a project using decorative letters, etc.

So how do you come up with multiple topics for, say, a group collage? That is what this chapter attempts to explain.

Kick-start
We are creatures of habit: we tend to take the same route to work each day, and buy the same familiar brands of products. In fact we are on automatic pilot most of the time.

In our complex lives, this saves us having to learn everything from scratch each moment. But when this response becomes habitual, we gradually lose our alertness and curiosity - two traits that are prerequisite to thinking creatively .

During crisis situations or when being confronted with something unexpected, our preconceptions fall away and we become hyper-alert.

Think of three topics for an abstract collage to make together, (hint: blue things, squares, circles).

1 Mosaic. Light → dark

2 Shades of green

3

People often describe these moments as peak experiences where they feel more alive and are highly creative in their responses.

But to kick-start our creative brains we don't need a crisis situation, we can find other ways to break out of 'Seen this – done that' mode.

The first and simplest way is to become aware of how we use our attention, then learn to direct it in new ways. Our senses need to be sharpened so we can look, hear, smell, feel, and taste the world around us as if we were experiencing everything for the first time.

Once your senses are open to your surroundings, you begin to notice things that you normally might have passed by.

And as you develop your powers of observation your intuition will also develop.

All of these traits contribute to making you a more creative and responsive caregiver/companion because you become more alert and flexible in any situation.

The next section, *Tools for creative thinking* contains some ideas to help you to sharpen your attention, slow down and use your imagination.

Tools for
creative thinking

Getting into the creative mode

Pay attention

Slow down, look around. Take time generally to form sensory impressions.

The journey is as important as the destination

Walking from one building to the other can be a rushed dash or a moment to breathe and recharge one's batteries

Take the time to find out what your preferences are

Consider ignoring commercial trends and outer influences for awhile and home in on your own particular interests.
For example: on vacation, each person relates to a new country in a unique way. One prefers sampling the beaches and food. Another will familiarise herself with the landscape through walking. Someone else will visit the historic churches and museums, and still another will comb the shops, looking for a particular collectible or souvenir. What do you do?

Regularly expose yourself to new input

Consciously break habits; choose a book by an author you've never read, see the work of an unfamiliar artist, get to know someone who doesn't belong in your familiar circle of friends.

Learn to make connections between unrelated things.

Have you found an interesting piece of hardware in your garage? Make it an activity. Did you meet a new person with an unusual skill or occupation? Invite them to the nursing home to share it with the residents.

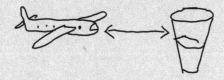

All of the following are close at hand and can be rich sources for activities:

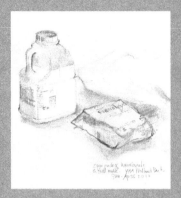

YOURSELF
your culture, family, stories, experience, work, and travels

IMMEDIATE ENVIRONMENT
history, anecdotes, local events, unusual landscape features

sketches from a travel journal

MATERIALS/OBJECTS
second hand, antique, recycled magazines, etc

FRIENDS
bring along someone with an interesting occupation and interview them, or let a storyteller, musician, poet or masseur share their skills

CATALOGUES
gardening tools, artworks (good for collage), hardware, car parts, clothing, furniture

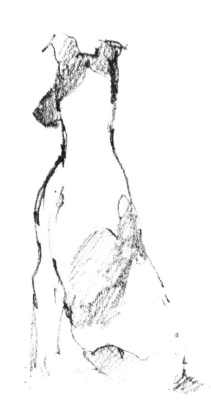

THE MOMENT
atmosphere, season, holiday, time of day, local events, historical events, other people

ENCOUNTERS/PEOPLE
previous encounters, their clothing, their mood, words, gestures

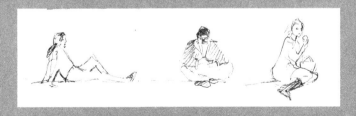

 **KEEPING AN** # IDEA NOTEBOOK

ONE WAY TO GENERATE IDEAS IS TO SAVE YOUR IMPRESSIONS IN A NOTEBOOK.

KEEP IT WITH YOU AND WRITE DOWN IDEAS AND EXPERIENCES AS THEY COME.

YOU CAN ALSO ADD QUOTES, IMAGES, etc. BY CUTTING THEM OUT AND PASTING THEM INTO YOUR NOTEBOOK.

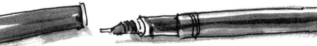

- FAVOURITE CALLIGRAPHY FOUNTAIN PEN

IT DOESN'T TAKE SIGNIFICANT EXTRA TIME.

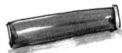

The book will eventually fill up with your unique impressions. Looking through it you will see previously vague ideas in a tangible form which can be reviewed, arranged, & changed.

THIS MATERIAL BECOMES A SOURCE FOR NEW IDEAS WHICH CAN SPILL OVER INTO OTHER AREAS OF YOUR LIFE

* Some of the quotes & sketches in this book came from my Idea notebooks

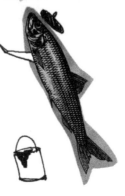

YOU CAN USE YOUR NOTEBOOK TO TRY OUT ALL KINDS OF DIFFERENT THINGS

YOU CAN KEEP YOUR NOTEBOOK PRIVATE OR SHARE IT. EITHER WAY KNOW THAT:

artists' and other creative thinkers journals are usually messy.

PERFECTION is not a requirement for CREATIVITY and can even inhibit *spontaneous* expression!

IF YOU BECOME INTERESTED IN A MORE VISUAL APPROACH

TRY RECORDING YOUR IMPRESSIONS THROUGH SKETCHING & COLLAGE. AND EXPERIMENT WITH DIFFERENT WAYS TO DRAW YOUR WORDS (or emphasise) SOME ARE SHOWN HERE.

DONDERDAG · THURSDAY · JEUDI 27

KEEPING AN IDEA NOTEBOOK IS AN EFFECTIVE TOOL FOR CREATIVE THINKING. IDEAS COME WHERE THERE IS ACTIVITY – EITHER WORK OR PLAY WILL START THE CREATIVE FLOW MOVING.

JUST START SOMEWHERE!

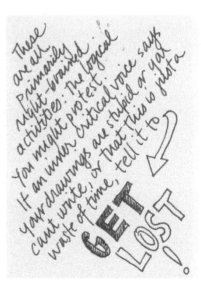

These are all primarily right-brained activities. The logical you might protest. If an inner critical voice says your drawings are stupid or you can't write, or that this is just a waste of time, tell it to GET LOST!

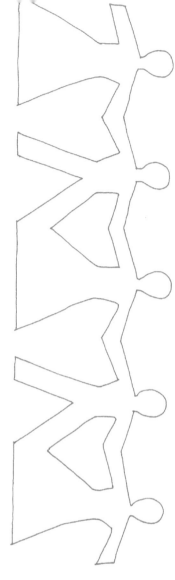

More ways to generate ideas
Start with one activity idea, for instance, making a paper doll.
Think up three variations.
Now think of ten more.

How to generate more ideas:

Variation
You could vary one or more elements, for instance: paint it
rather than colour in with pencils, collage the clothes, and
use different materials like washi rice papers to create
clothing textures.

Research
Use reference material to get ideas: national costumes
from different cultures, story book characters.
Go to a museum or gallery and look for clues to
new perspectives.
Browse art, hobby and budget shops for fun materials:
sequins, glitter, ribbons.

Change point of view
Think outside the box:

- ask an expert
in an unrelated field
for ideas

- engineer
- doctor
- carpenter

- change the
sex of the doll

`THE WAY
IT WAS
ALWAYS DONE'
BOX

- change the
species of the doll

- look at the
results of people
who did it 'wrong'-
'mistakes' can lead
to new ways of
seeing.
(see 'Samy')

- change the scale,
for example make it lifesized
from an outline of the
resident's body

Any kind of creative thinking is undertaken in the spirit of exploration without trying to control the outcome.

Usually these kinds of activities are accompanied by an attitude which asks, 'What if?'. What if I tried this or this? What would happen?

Also essential to creative thinking is learning to accept that making mistakes is a necessary part of the creative process. Often it is the mistakes, messes, 'failures' that break us out of the old way of thinking and force us into new territory.

If you get used to working and thinking in this way, your explorations will eventually connect with convictions or questions that are meaningful for you. And you will begin to create a body of thoughts and (visual) impressions that are entirely authentic. Most artists are in this mode all the time, and it enriches daily life in unexpected ways.

There are countless ways to develop your powers of creative thinking. Brainstorming, visualisation, and associative thinking are a few. Books and internet sites on developing your creativity are abundant. I'd rec-ommend Keri Smith's, 'How to be an explorer of the world' (2008), or 'Wreck this journal' (2007) to start you off.

See the end of this book for more information.

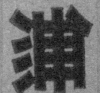

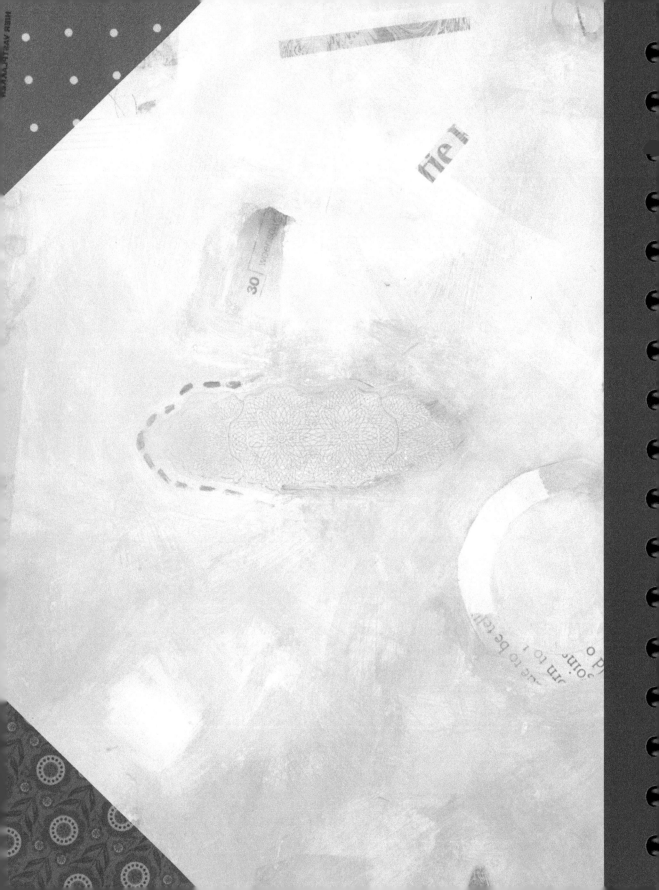

Activity basics, getting started

Sometimes it can be hard to know where to begin when there are so many ideas to choose from.

To help you narrow down the choice, I've cross-referenced much of the information in this book into several different mini-guides, each with their own categories, ideas and information. Please see the end of the book for the *Mini-guides* list (p176).

Preparing the activity

To choose an activity, you can either leaf through the book, refer to the *Activities list* (p180) or consult the *Mini-guides* (p176). Pick one easy activity that appeals to you and doesn't need too much preparation.

Read through the description of the activity and imagine going through it with the person you have in mind. Write your own notes if desired.

Then think of some back-ups (Plan B) if the person isn't in a condition or mood to do the activity that moment. (See mind map/chart, p63.)

When you arrive

Introduce yourself, greet the person, assess the situation, and decide if the activity is appropriate.

If you have, for example, planned to write down their thoughts during a conversation, begin the conversation. See where it leads, if it appears that the person isn't engaged, perhaps it would be better to go for a walk, continue the conversation on the walk, or switch to plan B.

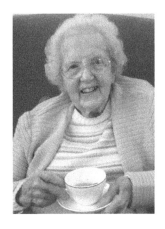

Duration

The activity can last as long as the person is interested and occupied. You may need to change the activity or the pace several times.

Remember, even five minutes of engagement is a success, and even one moment of lucid contact can completely change someone's day for the better.

Leave taking

Five to ten minutes before you need to go, warn the person that you will soon be leaving. Do this several times before you go. Begin to taper off the activity gradually, by starting to clean up materials, if necessary. Then gently disengage the person from what they are doing, and as clearly but gently as possible, leave. If the person is still occupied and you don't want to interrupt them, perhaps you can ask someone else to take over for you.

Note though, that the activity 'takes place in the space between you and the person' Byers (1995) so sometimes your absence can change or end the activity.

Evaluation

Review for yourself how the time was spent and what kind of feelings you observed in yourself and the other person.

Also note any points which were successful and others which were not.

For example:

Making a paper flower – the person was interested in the colour of the tissue paper but not in any hands-on activity. So maybe looking at magazine pictures and discussing colours, or making a collage based on a colour theme would be a more 'successful' activity. Or, if the person is unable to participate, you could make a bouquet of paper flowers for them – one or two each time you visit.

The chart to the right gives Plan B alternatives for an activity.

Original plan ➡ **CRAFT ACTIVITY**
MAKING A TABLE DECORATION

SITUATION 1

Person uninterested in activity but open to communicating

SITUATION 2

Person becomes fascinated with one detail of activity only

SITUATION 3

Person is sleepy and passive

PLAN B

1A or **1B**

1A: Sit with the person and do activity for or with them

1B: talk about the activity or a different topic

2A or **2B**

2A: fetch coloured felt pens or other drawing materials

2B: give pieces of paper to tear or crumple

3A or **3B**

3A: Listen to music or read together

3B: go out for a walk or a wheelchair stroll

FURTHER ENGAGEMENT

person does one small task

you record conversation as it happens

Person colours in a square or circle etc.

make a collage or assemblage

conversation or other form of contact

Could lead to full engagement

person receives their words as a poem

OUTCOME

person engaged in colouring activity

art work

pleasant time spent together

Materials and tools

The *Creating your own activities* and the *100 activities handbook* sections contain a lot of visual art activities. I've tried to keep the tool and material requirements as basic as possible so that the projects can be done without first having to obtain specialised materials. A pencil, paper, glue and scissors will bring you a long way with many of the projects in this book. Note: the g (grams) notation refers to the paper's thickness, not the quantity. 80g is normal white paper, 160g is heavier.

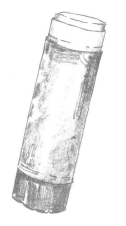

Here is a suggestion for a **basic craft kit** to either keep at the home or bring with you:

> 2 or 3 Pencils
> Scissors
> Stick glue
> Paper, coloured and white, light weight and card weight
> Origami papers
> Some coloured felt tips or coloured pencils

I store and transport my basic supplies in a large transparent cosmetic bag.

Below are **additional tools/materials** which can be useful to have on hand:

> Awl – for making holes in paper and cardboard. You can use a T-pin or dart point for this as well.
> Thin wire for making paper flowers
> Thick wire for mobiles
> An assortment of ribbons
> Coloured tissue paper for flowers and collages
> A compass
> Plastic craft cord or lanyard

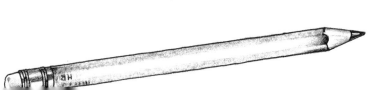

Masking tape
Embroidery threads
A selection of coloured card 160 gram A4
A selection of coloured paper 80 gram A4
Self adhesive decorative paper – silver, glittery or
   shiny coloured
Broad edged window or blackboard markers (washable)
Set of large-tipped felt markers for drawing

Low-cost-no-cost materials to collect:
Fabric scraps
Old magazines for collages
Jar lids for drawing circles
Collection of dried pressed flowers and leaves for collage
   and mobiles
Large wooden and glass beads from old jewelry
Flat, stiff clear plastic from packaging
Old cardboard boxes to cut up to use as patterns
Used wrapping paper and ribbons for collages
Old wallpaper and paint sample books for collage
Old CDs for mobiles – they catch the light nicely
Plastic bottle caps and pulls for the tactile exploration
   cord on page 114
Cardboard mailing tubes

Tips:
To make an individual whiteboard – go to a print shop and have
a white A4 (8 ½″ x 11″) 160 gram sheet laminated with thick
plastic. Buy a whiteboard marker and you have a mini whiteboard upon which people can draw. One wipe with a soft cloth
and the image is erased. If you want to preserve the image,
you can photocopy it.
See page 149 for a project using whiteboard.

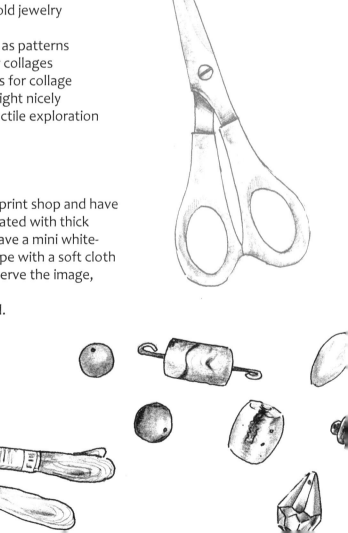

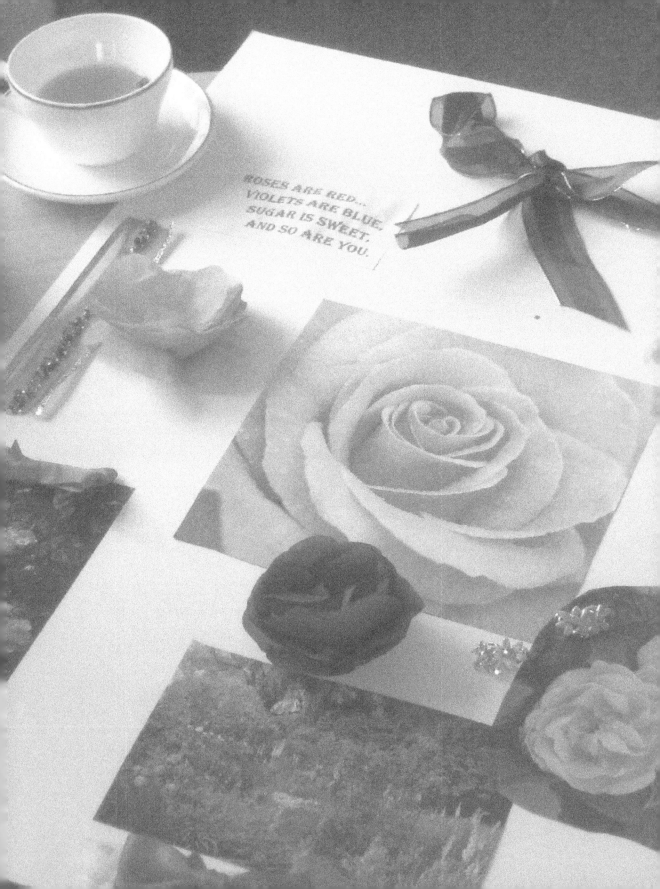

ROSES ARE RED...
VIOLETS ARE BLUE,
SUGAR IS SWEET,
AND SO ARE YOU.

3

CREATING YOUR OWN ACTIVITIES

Introduction to the activities section, doing the exercises

The following section is divided into ten chapters, each with a theme, for example: *Their story, history; Games and play; Cooking, food, and eating*, etc.

Since the purpose of this book is to encourage you to come up with ideas based on your unique situation, these chapters do not contain lists of activities. Instead there is a short introduction to the topic, and then an exercise section to get you thinking about activities for this particular category.

These exercises are the heart of this book and to gain the most benefit from it, I encourage you to do at least a few out of each list. Points from the list might inspire your own ideas, write those down too.

Tips on how to do the exercises

Brainstorming is an open way of thinking that admits all ideas for consideration, no matter how seemingly far-fetched. A brainstorming session is meant to generate a large amount of ideas in a short amount of time. Write what comes to mind quickly and without judging it.

Have plenty of scratch paper handy for this phase, you can always choose the best ideas later.

Working with two or more people creates a fertile ground for generating ideas.

Choose the topic and state it clearly, for example: 'What changes can be made to make mealtimes more pleasurable for the residents?'

Brainstorming guidelines

Throw out 'onto the table' everything you can think of without judgement. Later, it can be assessed for practicality, but at the start, the crazier it is the more chance of it leading to a really creative, out of the box idea.

Example of a list of ideas for the topic:
What changes can be made to make mealtimes more pleasurable for the residents?

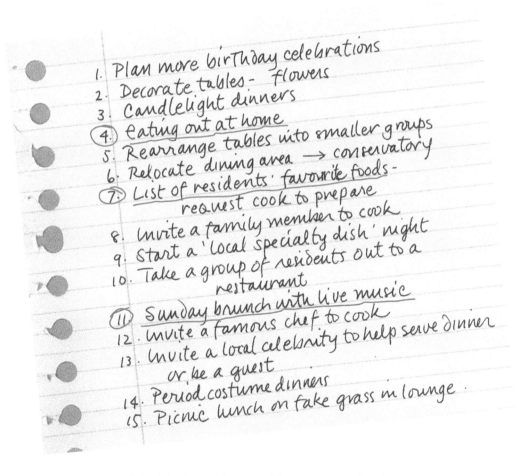

1. Plan more birthday celebrations
2. Decorate tables - flowers
3. Candlelight dinners
4. eating out at home
5. Rearrange tables into smaller groups
6. Relocate dining area → conservatory
7. List of residents' favourite foods - request cook to prepare
8. Invite a family member to cook.
9. Start a 'local specialty dish' night
10. Take a group of residents out to a restaurant
11. Sunday brunch with live music
12. Invite a famous chef to cook
13. Invite a local celebrity to help serve dinner or be a guest.
14. Period costume dinners
15. Picnic lunch on fake grass in lounge.

Choose a small doable list of the best ideas. You can further subdivide this list into 'long' or 'short term'.
If working with a group, decide who does what and when.

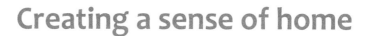

Creating a sense of home

I can imagine few things worse than being involuntarily uprooted from the safety and security of my home and placed in an institutional environment: to no longer be surrounded by familiar things, or to be able to putter in my studio, or just sit undisturbed dreaming in the sun.

What would you miss most if you had to leave your home for good?
Take a moment to consider the following: you have just come back from a weekend staying with friends and living according to their schedules and daily routines. What is the first thing you will do when you come back to your own home?
And what did you miss most? Was it the first cup of coffee enjoyed quietly at the start of the day? Was it your spouse or your children, pets or garden?

Especially for people in an institution these small losses adding up to a huge one must be addressed by providing a quality of attention that can help restore a sense of home, safety, and meaning.

A caregiver sensitised to the losses encountered when uprooted from home, family and neighbourhood will seek ways to compensate. Even the simplest engagements can make someone feel truly seen and cared for. I know from periods of illness, or other stress, that the presence of one kind person can make all the difference between feeling alone, and feeling connected and whole.

Here is a list of some losses that could be encountered when being removed from one's home and placed in an institution:

- Roles and status in the family and home, (provider, mother, cook, organiser)
- Roles in the neighbourhood (committee member, neighbour, babysitter, chairman of the club)
- Working roles
- Autonomy
- Privacy
- Intimacy
- Sex
- Pets
- Garden
- Hobbies
- Solitude
- Companionship
- Family events and trips

Think of ways you could help a resident recreate a sense of home. Are there ways to accommodate his schedule instead of the institution's? For example, see, *When is breakfast? Whenever you want!* (p77).
Involving a person in tasks such as meal preparation, waxing furniture, or caring for plants can restore a sense of meaning and purpose in their lives.

One care home doctor I spoke to encourages family and friends of the resident to continue on with normal activities, but to move these to the home when possible.
For example, one resident's bridge club continued to meet weekly, but in the lounge of the home. The resident could no longer play the game, but was included in the warm social event, the snacks, the joking and camaraderie.

Exercises

1   What easily made physical changes would create a sense of home? (Tip: a room screen or a curtain for privacy in shared rooms.)

2   A common problem in nursing homes is theft, as well as other residents simply wandering in and going off with personal belongings. Think up three ways residents could still be surrounded by familiar objects even when in a home. (Tip: anchor easily taken things to walls and tables.)

3   Create a 'day without' for a resident. Maybe they want to stay in their pyjamas or casual clothes. Maybe they would like to stay in bed all morning. Perhaps a woman would like to go without stockings or tight shoes.
What other things could they choose *not* to do?

4   Find out what a resident misses most, prompt with pictures, talk about the subject. And find ways to address this need. (Tip: bring a pet to be with, bring children to visit, take the person out more often.)

5   Think of five ways to better protect the resident's sense of privacy.
(Tip: knock on the door of their bedroom before entering. Always.)

6   Do you sense that someone is missing intimacy? If the nature of this is sexual, is there a way you could arrange for them to be alone with their partner somewhere away from the home?
If the person misses affection – cuddling, touching, and joking are easy to provide. List three ways to create more opportunities for intimacy.
(Tip: a luxurious bubble bath or a massage.)

7   How could you create more autonomy for the person? For example could they be put in charge of keeping supplies in order or answering a phone. Could they help another person, or tell staff if someone arrives or leaves? Could they have more choice in music, TV programmes, activities, or menus?

Special everyday moments

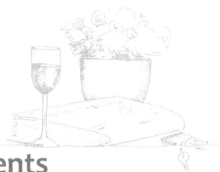

By removing people from their homes and neighbourhoods and placing them in institutional care our society takes away the normal roles, daily rituals and structure that give their days meaning; ironically this leads to 'activities' needing to be scheduled to fill up all that empty time.

Although special outings, in-house performances and other festive events are nice, we don't need to go to these lengths to create meaningful activity for someone.

Caregivers especially can add substantially to the quality of life of each resident by fully being with them and being alert to their needs.

By being fully present in your thoughts during the tasks you are doing, and by using your own creative resources, daily caring routines can become a real source of pleasure and engagement for both parties.

For example:
A caregiver knows she must get seven patients dressed by 10:00am.
She greets each person, senses their mood and current needs, asks them about their night, tells about her kids waking up early this morning. She takes two minutes extra to rub hand cream on Mrs C's hands, and her calm presence creates a circle of warm attention. She meets Mrs C's eyes and the old lady reaches out and touches the nurse's cheek, saying, 'Good girl'. The caregiver has similar moments with other patients, encounters very little 'difficult' behaviour, and ends up with the

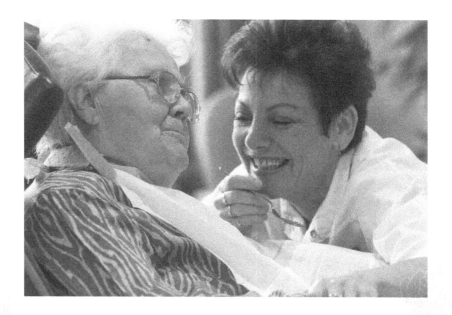

morning's tasks accomplished around 10:00am. She is feeling refreshed and nourished. Extra time spent: perhaps three to four minutes in all.

I know that every caregiver meets with unpleasant tasks and difficult behaviour, but very often the energy brought to an encounter influences how it will proceed, and the less stress the better.

Making ordinary moments special is creative, it is a way of being in and interacting with life which makes it repeatedly new. It is an alert, playful attitude that can be practised not just during work hours but all the time. This attitude opens up all kinds of possibilities for expressing yourself and at the same time caring more for the world and people around you. Things get less compartmentalised: you pick a flower on the way to work to give to a certain resident, or you buy a small antique doll at a flea market for a particular woman under your care.

What would happen if you brought your creativity to work with you every day? Here are some exercises to get you thinking in this direction. The keys here are 'simple' and 'low cost'.

Exercises

1 List three simple ways to decorate a breakfast tray or lunch table.

2 Think of three ways to make a make-up or shaving session extra special.

3 What could you talk about while dressing someone? (Hint: favourite colours, uniforms for different professions.)

4 Think of three ways to use aromatherapy oils to enhance someone's day.

5 How could you use music to enhance daily tasks?

6 Think of three ways to approach one of your most boring tasks in a different way. (Tip: fill a small spray bottle with water and add a few drops of rose or any other essential oil – this makes a natural room refresher.)

7 Bring nature closer through indoor gardening, walks, or cut flowers.

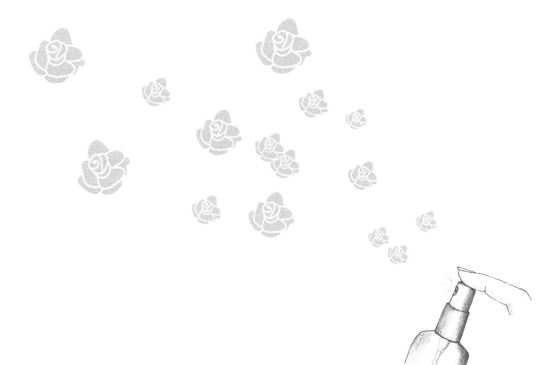

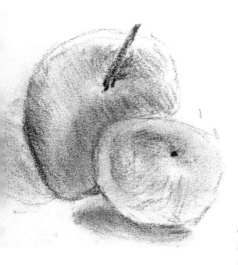

Cooking, food, and eating

Mrs M wasn't feeling well, and the staff told me she'd been refusing food and liquids for several days. Her bed had been rolled into the family room so she could have some company. That afternoon, the recreational director was preparing an apple pie. Everyone was gathered around a table sampling the apple slices and helping to press dough. I took a bite of apple and simultaneously got an inspiration. I went over to Mrs M and said, 'This is the most delicious apple I've ever tasted (it was), it is so beautiful and fresh, full of sunshine just like the day outside, I know you'll love it, please try it'. She seemed interested, but remained impassive, so I gently held a small piece to her lower lip to see if she would taste it. She opened her mouth and began to eat it.
I ate one, too, and gave her another. That disappeared as well as did the next two. When I left a little while later, she was sitting up, with colour in her cheeks.

The aim of all the ideas in this book is to normalise the life of a person with dementia at home or in an institution as much as possible. That is why, in the above example, it is important to note that the food was shared as a communal act rather than 'fed' as a form of physical maintenance.
A caregiver might not be able to share meals, but there is still a lot one can do to make the experience a shared and mutually nourishing one.

In one home I visited, the dining facilities were small private niches with seating for a maximum of six people. The feeling was much more 'restaurant' than institution. Coloured table-cloths, carpeted floors, beautiful chairs, filtered light through curtains, the presence of green plants, set the scene for a pleasurable and unhurried dining experience.

Another nursing home radically changed its approach in order to tailor meals to the needs of the residents rather than forcing residents to eat on the institution's schedule:

When is breakfast? Whenever you want!

During a seminar about the facility's philosophy, staff at a small nursing home agreed that they all embraced the idea of a people-oriented rather than task-oriented environment. However, they were concerned that these values were not being expressed in the daily routine of the home.

One particular nurse wondered why it was necessary to awaken residents early for breakfast when one of the things people look forward to when retiring is the freedom to get up and have breakfast when they want.

The staff were determined to create this kind of choice for the residents. This required a shift from an institutionalised- to a person-oriented schedule. The change demanded extensive cooperation and interdepartmental planning but the results were very positive.

Offering breakfast when the residents got up, instead of getting the residents up for breakfast resulted in: a less rushed staff, more relaxed residents, and a homey scent of coffee and toast in the home in the morning. An extra bonus which was structurally beneficial was the freedom from having to plan activities for the morning, since breakfast was an activity in itself. The project is now permanent. Zgola (1999).

To open the way for such creative change, attention first has to be given to habitual thoughts and routines which may be so ingrained as to be invisible. In the above example, nurses began to ask, 'What if breakfast didn't have to be served at a fixed time?' From the possibility of 'doing it another way', came a flow of energy and ideas to make it work. And from the willingness to make this happen, were born new routines that couldn't have even been imagined while still operating from within the old structure.

Food is a basic survival need. But it is also important socially. Mealtimes are when we come together with loved ones to talk about our day. Meals bring structure to daily life; they can be celebrations. With a little creativity, dining can be a truly nourishing experience for everyone involved.

Exercises

In a facility

1 How could you modify things in your care home to accommodate the residents' dining needs better? (Tips: location, time, content of meals, table setting.)

2 What is your favourite homemade food? What memories does it call up for you? Could you cook something to bring to the home and share your memories with the residents?

3 What regional specialties would the residents recognize? How could you work these into the menu?

4 Think up three safe ways to have a candlelight dinner (with or without real candles).

5 Think up five fun things to do with chocolate icing!

6 Find out the residents' favourite foods and get them.

7 Celebrate seasonal foods in four ways. (Tips: visually, taste, aroma…)

8 Make an easy cookie recipe together. Grade the activity so everyone can participate (see *Activity grading* p48).

9 Plan a High Tea for your group. Invite family to help and enjoy.

10 Is your facility multicultural? What rituals around food could you implement to make the meal an event? What elements could you apply on 'normal' days? (Tips: fresh spring flowers on the table or at each place, a silent meal, music, coloured serviettes, new seating arrangements, prayer, or a special guest.)

At home

All of the above can be adapted to make home mealtimes more pleasurable.

Is there another location you could try to eat in? (Tip: outside in summer.)

Is there someone you could invite over who would be welcome company (and tolerant of unconventional table manners) for the person with dementia and for you?

What would the person enjoy? (Breakfast in bed on a tray? Breakfast in front of the TV, or with music, going out together to a pub? Or taking a ride to pick up fish & chips?)

Menu

Croissants
Toast
homemade
Strawberry Jam
Cereal
Yogurt
Coffee, Tea
Herbal Tea

Making something for/with

The woman was completely immobilised by her diabetic condition and stared apathetically in front of her. I tried to get her involved in some simple crafts, but she declined.
So instead, I sat with her and started making a paper flower and while I worked asked about her life and interests.
One of her former hobbies had been handwork, but because of her illness and extreme overweight, she could no longer use her hands for exacting work. She could make some small movements, though, and from time to time I asked her to hold the glue for me, and once, to apply it. Soon she forgot her limitations and became totally involved. She made two flowers virtually without help. As I was leaving, a nurse came in and admired the flowers, she turned to the nurse and said emphatically,
'See, I can still do something!'

One way to spend time with someone is to engage in a creative activity in their presence. Depending on their abilities they can participate or just watch. Even if they cannot actively partici-pate, there are ways to involve them. See the chapter on *Activity Grading* (p48).

You can start by explaining what you are going to do and what the purpose is: 'I am going to make this flower to decorate your bulletin board and you can help me out if you like'.
You can involve them by asking questions related to the activity: 'Which of these is your favourite colour? Would you like to pick out one of these papers (pens, objects, images)?'

As you gain more insight into what the person is capable of, you will be able to gently prompt them to take over certain tasks. They can hold the glue or the scissors, they may be able to cut, paste or fold. You can do any of those movements together by placing your hand on theirs if appropriate, and they will still have a sense of having participated.

Even if they do nothing but watch, you can ask their opinion about certain steps.

If your attitude is one of enjoyment and inclusiveness, they will feel satisfaction when it is done, and will have been pleasantly occupied for the time that you've been working.

Try to find an area of common interest that you both will be inspired by. Make something functional or decorative for their room or the lounge. Make something with their name on it. Avoid projects that look like kindergarten art by selecting adult art products like beautiful handmade papers in subtle and rich colours. Avoid using only primary colours like yellow, red and blue. Set them off with deep purples, olive greens, hot pinks, greys and rust colours. Or use a selection of gradated tints, from a shell pink to a deep fuchsia in five steps. Cartridge paper is a borderline case, I've mostly avoided it but if you must use it, complement with shiny or glitter papers.

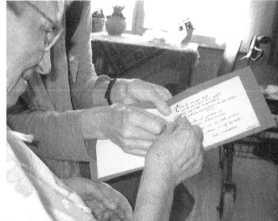

Remember, creative work imperfectly done is still a creative accomplishment, and sometimes art! The creative activity is a means not the end. The main purpose is to spend a companionable, constructive time and if there is a nice product at the end to show for it, that is a bonus.

In the past, I have entered a lounge filled with dozing residents and at the end of the afternoon left a group of energetic involved people. I would usually begin by going around and greeting people personally, while covertly assessing their energy and attention levels. I'd remind them why I was there and often would begin with a few individuals who had fairly constant activities.

Mrs F disliked any craft work but was happy with her enlarged crossword puzzle (see *Games and Play* p84). I'd sit with her while she started, then she worked solidly on her own for an hour or more.

Mrs G was very creative and made beautiful artworks from the prints of mandalas I brought for her. We would start out working side by side on different ones, and I would occasionally give a suggestion about colour or design if she seemed stuck. (See *Mandalas*, p162.)

Mr V would already be sitting at the table reading his paper, and could be drawn into a word or trivia game with a few other residents.

Several others would enjoy looking at picture books from the library, while a few more could be engaged in a simple craft activity like collage.

I was able to move around from person to person giving individual attention to 8-10 people for the full two hours I was there.
And even if there were some people simply sitting at the table enjoying everyone else's busyness, they became caught up in the general atmosphere. The pleasant sounds and signs of activity drew staff and visitors to come and see what was going on; sometimes they would be invited to join in.
The activity literally transformed the atmosphere in that part of the home for the whole afternoon.

Exercises

· ·

1   Look on the internet or at a hobby shop for easy to make paper flowers – these are no-fail and pretty. There are directions for some in *To make for the room* (p124-25).

2   Think of three topics for a theme collage to make together. (Hint: children, pets.)

3   Think of three topics for an abstract collage to make together. (Hint: blue things, squares, circles.)

4   Think of three topics for a group collage to do together around a table (Hints: local interest, seasonal.)

5   Find an easy origami form and learn it.

6   Simplify a hobby of yours and teach it to someone. (Hint: embroidery – make a design in a simple running stitch for them to follow.)

7   Design three activities around a hobby or profession of the individual. (Hint: dressmaker – bring in some nice fabrics, make a simple potpourri bag *To make for the room* (p119).

8   Use decorative letters (calligraphy) to personalize something for them. (Tip: name sign for their door, *Letters and handwriting* p142.)

Games and play

Most games involve complicated cognitive skills and so become difficult and frustrating for people in advanced stages of dementia. But that is no reason why these individuals should be denied the companionship, fun and sense of achievement playing games can bring. Especially people who have played card or other games most of their lives should be given the opportunity to enjoy this activity.

In his book, *Keeping Busy*, James R. Dowling (1995) devotes a long chapter to word games. One may ask, how could games involving memory and language be appropriate for individuals with dementia? But words, especially familiar phrases, sayings and expressions stay in the brain for a long time. I have played a number of games involving words and memory with people with varying degrees of dementia and they have been surprisingly successful.

Modifying games

One way to use your creativity in this area is to modify existing games to the level of cognitive ability of the person you are working with. Think of the game as a way to spend time in companionship, and also to provide the chance for the individual to gain a sense of achievement. Winning or losing as goals are replaced by personal accomplishment.

There are some individuals, for example, who continue doing crossword puzzles for a long time despite other cognitive difficulties. One woman had stopped this familiar activity because her eyes were failing her; when I enlarged the puzzle on the copier, she was able to enjoy doing them again. As she began to find them increasingly difficult because of the advance of the disease, I sometimes gave her blanks of ones she had completed, and these were easier for her. I allowed myself this small subterfuge because it so obviously enforced her self-esteem. If she commented that one seemed familiar, I said, 'Yes, we might have done this one already, several months ago', and she was fine with that.

When I caught sight of a box game of, 'Memory' in the activity room of the psychiatric nursing home where I worked, I was surprised to learn that it was regularly used with people with dementia.

Game play: The goal is to discover matching pairs. The deck of cards is shuffled and the cards are laid face down in a grid. Players take turns turning two cards at a time face up. If there is no match, the cards are returned to their face down position. Meanwhile the players try to memorise which they were and where in the grid they were located. The next player turns over two more cards, keeping in mind the cards revealed in the previous player's turn. The game progresses until someone turns over a matched pair, she removes them from the grid and keeps them and gets another turn.

Some people in early stages of the disease could remember and match the pairs of cards, but I was curious how one would use the cards with people who had lost those abilities. So I explored ways to use the cards as a starting point for games which were suited to each person's level of ability. Almost any simple (card) game can be adapted in this way. For example, with 'Memory', if the person can't remember the position of the card she just turned over, instead of returning the card to its face-down position, you can leave the card exposed until she finds the match.

Try out some of the exercises following to develop your own ideas for fitting games to abilities, and see the chapter *Activity grading* (p48).

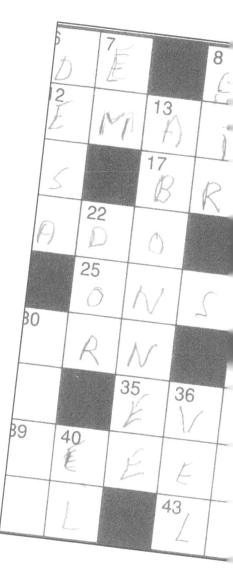

Mrs S has filled out this crossword puzzle perfectly. In her native language – Dutch.

Exercises

1   Think up three variations of 'Memory' that still depend on retaining the positions of the cards, but have fewer elements to keep track of. (Tips: smaller choice, non-competitive, involving movement or sound.)

2   Now, using the same cards create three games that are not dependent upon memory. (Tips: categorise the images by colour, for example; sort; arrange.)

3   Quartet or Happy Families game combined with personal history:

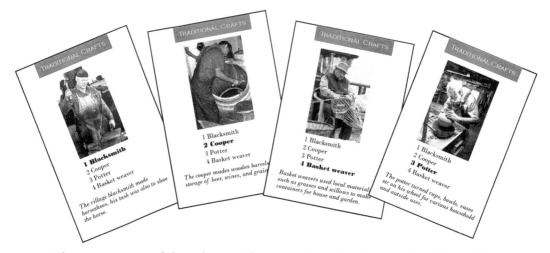

The most successful card game I've ever played with people with moderate cognitive impairment was a quartet game based on local regions – the neighbourhoods and era in which the residents had grown up. The cards were a generous postcard size and contained sets of drawings (four to a set, you could use photos instead). They were divided into categories: *Famous landmarks, Old occupations, Regional food specialities, Illustrations of dialect expressions and sayings, Clothes,and Household items.*

Everyone present was engaged, and those who had no grasp of the 'game' were drawn easily into discussion about each topic revealed on the cards.

Make your own regional quartet game based on the area where most of the residents came from, or the region or country.

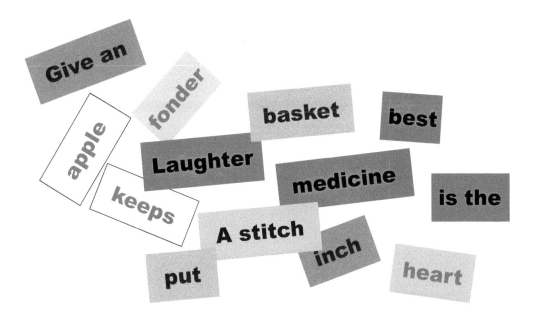

4   Another successful and easy game to make is 'Sayings'. Familiar proverbs are printed on heavy coloured paper, laminated with clear plastic, then cut into fragments and shuffled.
The goal of the activity is to re-assemble the fragments so that they form a complete proverb.

Familiar sayings are so ingrained, they seem to be less subject to loss when memory starts to break down. 'A stitch in time…' can be easily completed by many people with dementia.

Think up a mode of play for each of the four levels below:
 a People who can still read and comprehend what they are reading.
 b People who can read but need help in interpreting what they have read.
 c People who can't read but can recognize and complete the sayings verbally.
 d People who can't participate at a cognitive level but enjoy arranging things.

Their story, history
reminiscing and identity

People who have dementia are fully mature adults with a lifetime behind them. Most of them have raised children and held responsible positions at work.

When placed into institutional care they are not only threatened with the loss of their functions in their immediate neighbourhood and community, but also their roles as directors of their own lives.

Every effort should be made to support the autonomy and identity of people with this condition. Being genuinely interested in the person's past is an effective way to do this and it can be a great gift to both of you: the person gets the opportunity to tell you about it, and you get to learn more about an era gone by.

For me, an American living in the Netherlands, it has been especially enlightening to learn about the history of the area we live in, from how people cleaned carpets before vacuum cleaners (they dragged the rug out in the winter and cleaned it with snow), to what was sold in the earliest grocery stores (loose herbs, grains and sugar scooped into triangular folded brown bags).

Communicating creatively

Despite the fact that someone who is cognitively impaired may have trouble communicating and understanding speech, he is still the most important person to ask about his life.

There are creative ways to enable the person to communicate who they are and what they need even if they are in later stages of the illness.

In Israel, for instance, a team travelled around to institutions to collect profiles of residents, not from the staff, but from the residents themselves. They did this by sitting around a table and showing a selected few people pairs of adjectives one at a time. The individuals were asked to choose which one would describe them best. 'Even severely cognitively impaired people were able to provide a fairly complete profile of themselves.' Zgola (1999).

In Scotland, social workers have used evocative words on cards with the residents to form accurate evaluations of the care they were receiving. Killick J (2003).

Getting to know me

In my own work at the nursing home, I adapted Zgola's (1999) *Getting to know me* page (originally designed for use at admission meetings) into an activity.

The goals of this activity were to confirm and support each person's identity and to remind family and carers that they were dealing with whole, valid people. And there was much enjoyment for everyone in collecting the information.

A description of that activity follows.

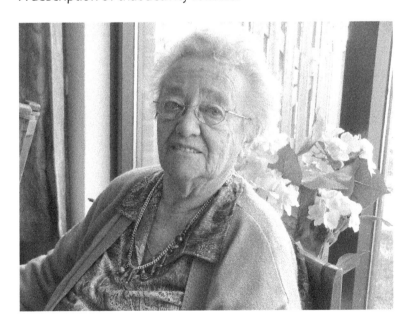

GETTING TO KNOW ME

MY NAME IS *Mrs. Richard Faber*

MY NICKNAME IS *Marti*

I WAS BORN IN (Place) *Groningen, NL*

FOR MOST OF MY LIFE I LIVED IN *Leens*

MY OPINION ABOUT THAT PLACE WAS *OK, considering our difficult family situation*

MY FAVOURITE HOBBY IS/WAS *sewing & knitting*

THE PERSON IN MY LIFE WHO INFLUENCED ME THE MOST WAS *hard to say*

BECAUSE, *... no answer*

MY FAVOURITE FOOD IS *meatloaf*

MY FAVOURITE SPORT IS *gardening and cycling*

MY FAVOURITE LOCATION IN THE WHOLE WORLD IS *Holland*

IF SOMEONE WERE TO TELL YOU THE BEST THING ABOUT ME THEY WOULD SAY *I am a good mother*

MY BEST CHARACTERISTIC IS *good mother*

UP UNTIL NOW THE THING I AM MOST PROUD OF IN MY LIFE IS *my son, and I have 2 daughters and seven grandchildren!*

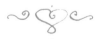

GETTING TO KNOW ME

Preparation
I wrote out the questions (see next page) for myself and numbered them, leaving several blank spaces between each question to write the answers in.
Then I made several copies: I wrote the name of each resident at the top of one of the copies and used that to record the information of each resident.

The Session
I worked my way down the question list either individually, one to one, or with a group.
The group sessions were lively and productive, as people opened up more as the session progressed.

I found that if family members were present, they sometimes contradicted the resident's answers; occasionally I opted to write down the resident's responses, since they were poetic and often revealed more about themselves than the family's more logical explanations.

Example:
  Question: 'What was your favourite sport?'
  Resident's answer: 'Ice skating'.
  Daughter: 'Mother never ice skated, she played tennis'.
  Resident: 'I always loved skating on the canals in
  the winters'.

The collecting of information proceeded at each individual's pace, and could take a half an hour or more in a group. Next, I read everyone's answers back to them, with much hilarity from the group. However, there were also moments of being genuinely moved by someone's story.

To conclude. I thanked everybody and promised them they would each receive a copy to hang up in their rooms.

At home, I made up an attractive document to honour each person. See page to the left.

I wanted it to resemble a diploma and act as acknowledgement for a unique life lived.

I added extra interest and value by filling the answers in calligraphy.
Any kind of legible fancy or coloured writing would do.

I had the final document laminated in heavy plastic, but you could also frame it.

THE QUESTIONS

My name is

My nickname is

I was born in

For the most of my life I lived in

My opinion about that place was

My favourite hobby is/was

The person in my life who influenced me most was

My favourite food is

My favourite sport is

My favourite location in the whole world is

If someone were to tell you the best thing about me they would say

My best characteristic is

Up until now the thing I am most proud of in my life is

You can tailor the questions for groups or individuals, or spread out the questioning over several sessions to get a more balanced picture of the person. You could choose different themes for each session. See this chapter's *Exercise* section.

BACK TO NOW BOOK

The *Back to Now* book is a further development of *Getting to Know me.*
During the time I worked with people with advanced dementia, I developed this as an ongoing project to honour and celebrate each individual. It was simply a loose-leaf 2 ring binder with various sections. I called it *Back to Now* because it was a way to save moments, to save the 'now', and revisit them.

The categories were:
> **Getting to know me**
> **Outings**
> **Writings**
> **Art**
> **Visitors book**
> **Other**

Getting to know me
A filled in questionnaire designed to tell more about the person than meets the eye.
See previous section in this chapter.

Outings
A place for staff and families to paste pictures and short descriptions of outings that the person had participated in, but had often forgotten the next day.
A related activity would be to go through this section and reminisce about the trip to the zoo or the boat tour. Often the person wouldn't remember the specifics but would remember the emotions associated with the festive day.

Writings
I always wrote down snippets of conversation, sometimes making them into poems. This form of cooperative creative writing is described in the next category. By keeping the results in the book, the person eventually became very impressed with what they had written. And it was a new perspective for family and caregivers who had not suspected these sorts of depths in the person.

One of the related activities was to then decorate the poem using collage, stamping, or other visual art techniques.

Art

All the A4 format pages containing drawings, paintings, or collages were kept in this section. The most popular form of art was colouring in mandalas (p162). One woman had a beautiful colour sense and adored going through her book, looking at her completed work and showing it to others.

Visitors Book
Sometimes a resident would be distressed waiting for a visit that had already taken place. In one instance, a woman waiting for her brother to come, became increasingly agitated when caregivers told her that he had already been to see her yesterday. She was momentarily aware that she had lost that entire slice of memory and became angry with the caregiver for 'lying to her'.
Perhaps if the brother had written a message plus the date of the visit in the book, this might have calmed her. However, it is also possible that she might not have understood this either, or may not have accepted it because it would be proof that there was something wrong with her memory.

Nevertheless, a visitor's book can be helpful, especially if different family members from far off places regularly visit. I saw a book in which the four daughters of one woman recorded details of their visits with their mother. They included what they had done with their mum that day, her health and appearance, and things she had said.

Other
This is a catch-all for other material pertinent to the person's identity. For example a particularly meaningful letter could be taped in this section, or birthday cards or another form of award or appreciation. I included objects found on walks, pressed flowers, crosswords or other puzzles completed, etc.

Exercises

1. Think of three themes for *Getting to know me* sessions.
   (Tips: music, hobbies, etc).

2. What interest of yours could coincide with something from the person's past? For instance, as a calligrapher, I wanted to know how they learned to write. I brought in old pens and inks to jog their own memories of learning to write.

3. If you were in a nursing home, what objects now would then be antique (say, 30 years from now). What objects do you think would hold particular nostalgia for you?

4. What antique object could you bring in for them to start up reminiscences?
   (Hint: vintage food- or sweet tins.)

5. What piece of music could you bring for a resident to bring back old times?

6. Think up three topics to reminisce about concerned with 'home'.

7. Think up three topics to reminisce about concerned with work. (Tip: office, construction, restaurant, etc).

8. Think up three topics to reminisce about concerned with travel.

Collaborative creative writing

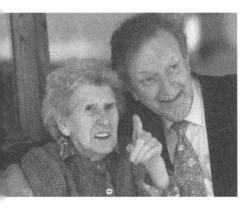

Giving time and attention to an individual, listening carefully to what they say tells each person with dementia that they are valued, that they are of interest and worth.

The further step of writing down what is said powerfully underlines that statement of worth. For the person with dementia this is a rare, maybe unique experience. John Killick's confidence in people's ability to communicate (even those who are severely damaged) has been rewarded with communications of clarity and intensity from people who care staff thought could hardly talk at all.

– Sue Benson, Foreword to *You are Words* (Killick 1997)

When I first heard about John Killick's pioneering work in writing poetry with people with dementia, it fired my imagination so much that I immediately contacted him. He graciously agreed to a visit and I flew to Scotland to meet with him at the University of Stirling: he was then director for creative projects and dementia care there.

John is a poet and writer so has developed particular skills as far as working creatively with words. But given a special kind of attention and an open creative attitude, anyone can do this work.

John creates poetry from the conversations he has with the individual. He does not alter their words, he either uses the words as they were said or at the most pares down what is said to the bare lines of thought.

Assessing verbal abilities

It will be up to you to assess the verbal abilities of the person. Be subtle and observe whether they are able to read and if they understand what they are reading. For instance,
you may ask for help in deciphering some printed words, and ask them about the meaning. Often people who have trouble formulating sentences can understand spoken words much better than they can speak them.
Whilst doing this work try to remove distractions such as radio and TV from the environment.

The procedure

When I have acted as a scribe for individuals with dementia, I recorded the conversation and arranged some of the longer lines into shorter more poetic phrases, for example:

'It was a house on the water just after Kantens almost to Rottum. Our factory was also on the water's edge, but it isn't there anymore'.

becomes:

> *It was a house*
> *on the water*
> *just after Kantens*
> *almost to Rottum.*
> *But*
> *it isn't there*
> *any more.*

The main point is that the voice of the speaker is not only kept intact but is actually amplified by how you arrange their words. The effort is certainly a joint one, but the voice remains that of the person who spoke the words.

The poem above takes the meaning of the words, which are quite rational and descriptive, at face value. 'Our family had a house' means exactly that.

But often the communication is less rational and this is where your imagination comes in.

I feel that my background in the ups and downs of creative work might have helped to develop a tolerance for irrational speech as well as appreciation for seemingly absurd use of language.

These unconventional uses of words are valid efforts to express and I treat them that way rather than trying to correct someone's language (unless they ask). If I don't understand the literal meaning then I try to sense the meaning underneath. And if I still don't understand, I tell them that the fault is mine.

When you look at words beyond their obvious meaning, a new context arises and there are several different levels you can work from:

All fragments below are from the book, *You are Words*, Killick (1997).

Poetic meaning and imagery of the words

Fragment from the poem, 'You are words':

>*I want to thank you for listening.*
>*You see, you are words.*
>*Words can make you or break you.*
>*Sometimes people don't listen,*
>*They give you words back,*
>*And they're all broken, patched up*

Poetic qualities- cadence repetition

Fragment from, 'Bell lane':

>*Tell tale Tit*
>*Your tongue shall be split*
>*And all the dogs in town*
>*Shall have a little bit.*
>
>*Where will we run to?*
>*Up Bell lane.*
>*I'll tell the teacher*
>*And you'll get the cane.*

Or: fragment from, 'Problems':

> *Are you sure there's nothing there?*
> *Well it must have been in another room.*
> *Well it must have been in the other house.*
> *Well it must have been another skirt.*

Words as symbolic expression of mood or idea

Fragments from, 'Home':

> *That door's squeaking. It hasn't very much sense.*
> *It makes you wonder who's looking after it.*

....

> *I think it is a pity to have all these people together in here.*
> *They don't wear as well as they would outside*

Words as art

Words for their own sake – nonsense to us, but expressing something totally individual.

Here is a fragment from, 'Writing it down':

> *You don't see your family*
> *much now: like a carrier bag*
> *on your back, one way or another.*
> *But you can't barge it or dish it-*
> *All of it was everwell.*

Presentation

Once you have written the words down, a further step is to present the results in some way. If you are an activities organiser or staff member, writing or printing out a poem or conversation can be a gift for the family; it shows you value the person as he is now. It could help the relatives see their loved ones in terms of what is still possible rather than loss. It might stimulate them to write memoirs of the person as well.

For directions on making the simple presentation booklet shown here, see *Poetry writing* in the *100 activities handbook* section (p129).

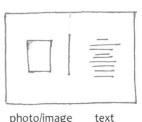

photo/image   text

Exercises

1 Reminisce with someone, write down what they say and turn it into a poem. (Tips for topics: old grocery store, farm, lakes, rivers, trips.)

2 How could you become someone's scribe? If you had dementia and could not write but were aware there were things you wanted to say, what would you want someone to write down for you and how would you let them know? Write three ideas for an activity around this topic. (Tip: a letter to a friend.)

3 Next time you go on a vacation, send a postcard to a resident. Think of three things you would need to do to make it understandable and that it is from you. (Tip: a sketch or cartoon about something you both have shared.)

4 How could you use words in combination with music? (Tip: a simple song or rhyme.)

5 What skill or hobby do you have which could enhance their words that you've recorded in writing? (Tip: calligraphy, decoupage, desk top publishing, photography.)

6 Poetry writing for elders, (see *100 activities handbook* p129).
 a. Write three poems yourself, using the tips from poetry writing for elders.
 b. Then write three poems with a person with dementia, using the same tips.

'Holding', and physical objects

You may be confronted, as I was, with people who are too far progressed in the disease to be able to comprehend any consecutive sequence of actions, much less grasp the end goal of such activity.

Instead they may do 'strange' things like try to eat art materials or hide their food in books or furniture.

What we need to remember is that these actions carry some kind of meaning for the person. Even if what they do is incomprehensible to us, we can still use the gesture (or sound or language) as a positive lead to support the person where they are.

This is achieved by a subtle shift from interpreting the action literally to using the action, when possible, as the basis for a creative engagement.

For example:

Mrs J had been a seamstress. She was a fastidious lady who refused to participate in any activities. When presented with sewing materials she would look mildly interested, but put them aside when prompted to 'do' anything with them.

I began bringing her different types of cloth to handle, and I put scissors and needles within her reach. When left to explore the materials on her own terms, she did become occupied. Once she wrapped a needle in so much yarn that it became completely hidden. She did this with an air of secrecy and hid the object when I came to look at it. (See photo p103.)

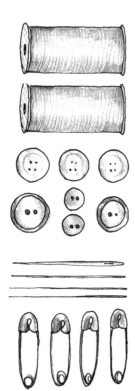

She also seemed to take pleasure in lining up the sewing materials on the table, though she didn't 'use' them in the usual manner.

Here you can see that the emphasis in these activities shifts from 'completing a task' or 'making something' to free exploration and manipulation of material as an end in itself.

To further this type of engagement you can provide a variety of materials to hold, wrap, cover, hide, pick up, examine, taste, and explore. Even the room can be a subject for interaction such as pushing against walls, or pulling at closed doors. These actions can be considered valid activities, as can becoming absorbed in the process of arranging and playing with objects in a way which indicates that this has meaning for the person.

Holding

Important in being with someone engaged in this type of action is an attitude called 'holding'. This is a non intrusive yet involved and aware presence.

Your role might be as an observer, or you may be invited to participate by being given an object or a meaningful look. Your powers of play, spontaneity and improvisation will be called upon.

Whatever takes place while the person is exploring or arranging happens in the context between you and the person.

For example, if you give Mrs S a pile of materials to look through it would not be appropriate, once having initiated the activity, to then leave the room – even if she seems oblivious of you.

Sometimes insights into the person can be gained from observing these interactions, but the goal of these activities is not directly therapeutic or diagnostic. The goal is to provide personal attention whilst the individual is engaged in meaningful and pleasurable activity.

Exercises

1 List ten different types of soft materials to explore and arrange.
   (Hint: cloth scraps, bubble pack.)

2 List ten different types of hard materials to explore and arrange.
   (Hint: smooth stones, wooden blocks.)

3 Name three shops where you could buy inexpensive materials to hold and
   explore. (Hint: ironmongers, interior decorating supply shops.)

(For safety reasons, when thinking of objects to use, assess first whether the
individual is prone to putting things in their mouth or might cut themself
with a sharp object).

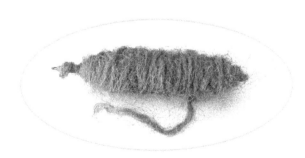

Start where they are
Activities based on hand movements and other gestures

In my wing at the home, there were several people who were no longer able to converse, comprehend, or interact in ways that I could understand. Armed with my box of materials, sometimes I could only watch while they did what to my eye were inexplicable things.

The departure points for activities in this section developed out of my ongoing exploration of how to engage these individuals on their terms. Rather than attempting to distract them from what they were doing, I tried to intuit what the significance of their actions might be. Why, for example, was Mr B tapping the arm of his chair incessantly? Was he trying to communicate? Mr B's tapping could signify impatience, why might that be? Once it was clearly linked to him desperately needing to use the toilet.

A logical cause/effect was not always evident; then I would respectfully enter into the moment with the person and build on their gestures or sounds. For instance, I might tap on the table in the same rhythm as Mr B, or try another rhythm. Or I might offer him a wooden dowel to use as an instrument.

Mrs G doesn't speak; she wipes the table in front of her repeatedly, back and forth, back and forth.
In my informal moments with her, I used her movements as the basis for several activities:
> *a. I gave her different textured cloths to wipe her table with and stayed with her while she tried them out, (appreciated).*

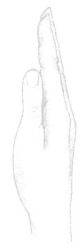

b. *Plastic toys and other obstacles were put on the table (angrily dispensed with in one powerful stroke).*

c. *Sat across from her and gently mimicked the wiping movements (no response except to occasionally try to move my hand away from what was clearly her table).*

d. *Put hand on hers and wiped together (sometimes allowed, sometimes ignored, sometimes withdrew hand).*

All of these moments are valid engagements which accept the person as she is with neither labeling nor trying to change the original behaviour.

Here are some common gestures I observed over the years I worked with people with dementia in nursing homes:

Tapping, patting
Stroking
Pressing
Pulling
Open hand
Grabbing, grasping
Folding
Rubbing
Rolling
Winding
Wrapping
Waving, swaying

This topic is further worked out in the *100 activities handbook*, (p166) but you might want to try the exercise below first.

- Select three gestures from above and think of several activities for each.

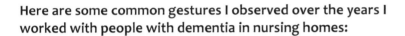

Witnessing-
when you can't *do* anything

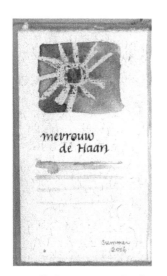

Detail of my memory book

During my first months working at the home, I encountered a disproportionately large percentage of people in the last weeks of their lives. At first I was at a loss, because there was not much one could do. But over time I found that just being there with the person could be a comfort to them, and to me as well.

Creative gestures

Since five people on the ward died in the first six months I worked there, I felt the need to mark these deaths in some way. I started a memory accordion book (p137). I commemorated each individual with a visual personal memory, either drawn or collaged. During the four years I worked there, many people passed away and I was able to remember each person's uniqueness and the gift of knowing them by giving them a page in my book.

I feel this was an important part of coming to terms with difficult and often distressing situations. And I believe creative gestures like this could be helpful in aiding caregivers to 'give a place' to the deaths they must experience regularly.

Witnessing

And admittedly, sometimes all you can do is 'witness'. It is an active gesture of accepting what is without trying to do anything about it.

You can sit near the person and hold their hand, or if you have a more intimate relationship with them, stroke their arm or cheek or hair. You can gently sing a song to someone or play an instrument softly. You can tell a story, you can pray together or meditate.

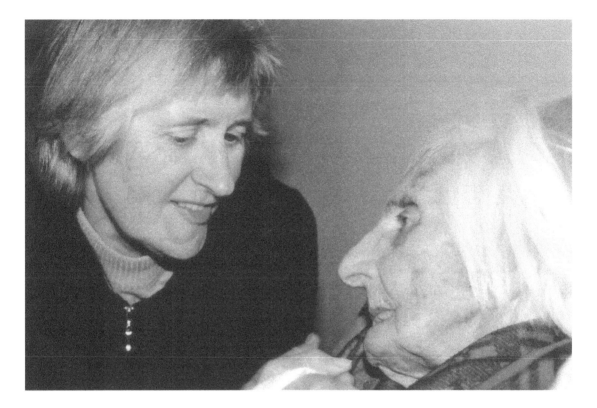

Creating order and beauty in the room is a way to be there;
even if the person seems not to be aware of, it is still an
appropriate and comforting way to show caring.

Snoezelen is a Dutch term which is now universally used to
refer to gentle sensory stimuli like bubble lights, soft music or
light projected on walls.
Whether these kinds of stimuli are appropriate or not depends
on the person's background and their present state. Some
people may find them relaxing, and others may simply find
them irritating, and let you know by agitated sounds or
movements or turning away.

Music, to the person's taste, played softly could be
appropriate.

Sometimes the presence of a peaceful dog can be comforting.

You can bring something to do with your hands that occupies only a part of your attention. Sit with the person and do sewing, small repair work, or clean out a drawer. Keep part of your attention free to speak softly with them, or be present silently.

I've sat quietly with many patients during their last hours on earth. Being there fully with someone, even if they are in pain or other distress is a profound way to witness and care at the same time.
A powerful practice is to match your breathing rhythm to theirs. John Killick and Kate Allan have documented their work with this method in the *Journal of Dementia Care*
(Killick J, Allan K 2005).

By being there as a witness, with or without words, you communicate to the person that they are not alone, and that they are valued. Sometimes this is all we can do.

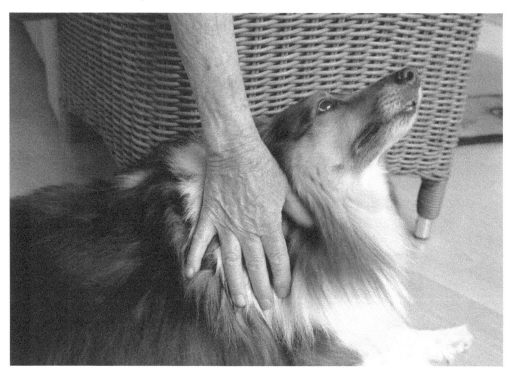

Exercises

1 How do you feel about just being there with someone without doing anything? If this is uncomfortable for you, list three reasons why. (Hint: 'I am getting paid to DO something, not just sit around'.)

2 Referring to the three reasons you might be uncomfortable with just sitting with someone, list three things you could do to be more comfortable in this situation. (Tip: remedies for this discomfort – sometimes just keeping someone company can make them feel good.)

3 List three things you could do to make the (institutional) room more pleasant. (Tip: make and hang a mobile with greeting cards received, see p120.)

4 Is there a roommate who makes noise and disturbs the individual you take care of? List three ways to remedy or modify this. (Tip: music, earplugs, room screen.)

5 List three ways to provide music for the person who is bedridden in an institution where things like a personal stereo player often 'disappear'. (Tip: bring a friend who sings or plays an instrument.)

6 Do you know someone who has a skill that would be pleasurable for someone who is bedridden? Invite them to visit. (Tip: alternative healing or massage.)

7 What skill would you like to learn to ease the person's discomfort or give them a pleasant experience? (Tip: see question 6)

8 List three small easily taken steps you could make to learn one of these skills. (Tip: look up what massage courses are offered locally.)
   a. Today
   b. This week
   c. This month

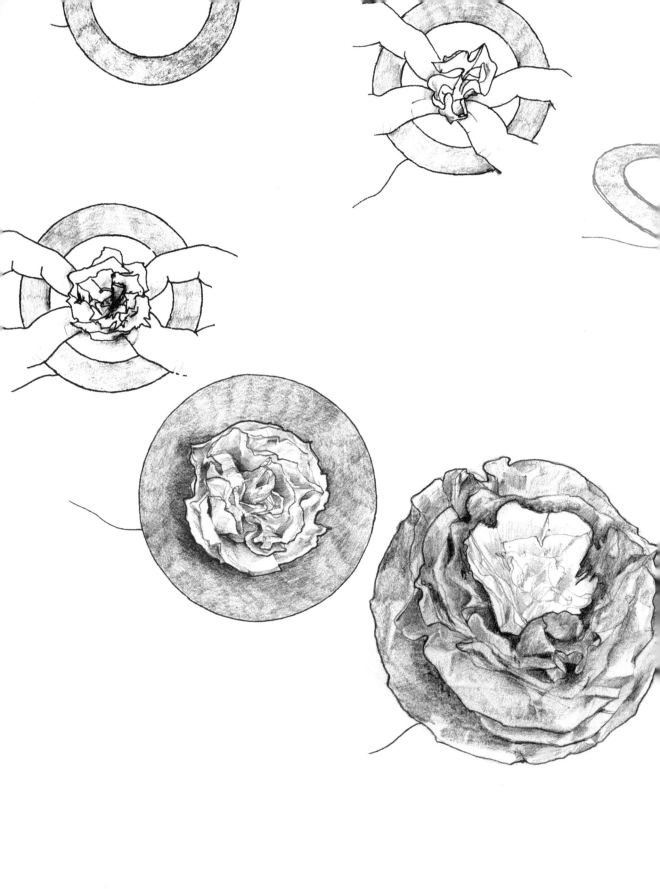

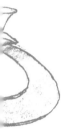

4

100 ACTIVITIES HANDBOOK

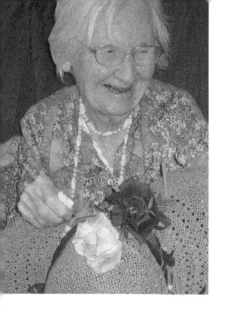

Introduction to the 100 activities handbook

If you have worked through the book more or less systematically and arrived at this point, you should now have a good foundation for developing and leading your own activities. You have hopefully learned about your own capacity for creative thinking and been able to experience the satisfaction of putting this into action. You will have been introduced to methods for grading activities, staying involved during simple actions, supporting the person where they are and more.

If you have jumped to this section to find ideas, I would suggest first reading the chapter on a creative approach (p16).

The previous section, *Creating your own activities*, contained exercises prompting you to think up your own ideas in a number of general categories.

This section, the *100 activities handbook*, provides you with lists of specific activities accompanied by step by step illustrated instructions.

The activities in this section may initially appear too difficult for people with dementia to complete. But that is not their primary purpose. Making something beautiful or functional (or both!) is a pleasant and active way to keep someone company. If they become interested enough to help a little, the activity engages them further. And if they actually become occupied with the subject or materials, the benefits, such as increased self-esteem, are even greater. (Also see *Activity grading* p48 and *Purpose and characteristics of activities* p40.)

A note about the measurements used in this book:

Sizes are given in centimetres and inches.

In Europe A4 is the standard page size used for printing, copying etc. In the USA, 8 ½˝ x 11˝ is used. In this book they are interchangeable even though they vary slightly in size.

Paper thickness is indicated in grams (g). 80g is standard printing and copying weight and 160g is a heavier card. 120g is in between and easier to fold than 160g.

No cost, low cost activities and exploratory material

The simplest ideas can be the most effective and they don't have to cost much. The examples following are tactile and visual tools/games which invite exploration.

One of the most effective 'table top games' I ever made was to string found objects on a lanyard cord. A certain woman in my group played with hers for hours, talking to it and not letting it out of her sight. She was eventually transferred to another home several miles away, and when I visited her months later, she was still talking to her 'toy'. See *Tactile exploration cord* on the next page.

Many of these activities are designed to address more than one sense. This heightens the chance of engagement. For instance, the *Tactile exploration cord* is primarily visual and tactile, but the clacking together of the CDs or bottle tops adds a sound element. The *Discovery tube*, too (p115), incorporates sound as it can be shaken like an instrument to rattle the contents.

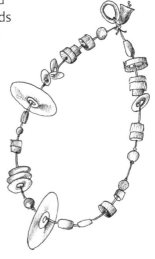

This multi sensory aspect is a good thing to keep in mind when thinking up your own ideas or working with the ones in this section.

MATERIALS

hole punch (usually used
  in leather work)

different sized plastic
  bottle caps (from
  juice, cooking oil etc)

large wooden beads

wooden rings

plastic or nylon cord, or
  lanyard (± 1½m, 1½ yds)

old CDs

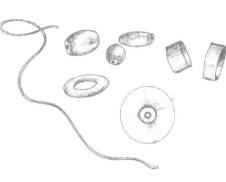

TACTILE EXPLORATION CORD

1 Punch holes in the plastic caps, large enough to easily
  thread the cord through.

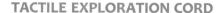

2 Take a length of cord, and begin to thread on the various
  objects. Some you will need to knot to keep in place, others
  you can let move freely along the cord.
  Alternate the open and closed surfaces of the caps.
  When you are finished, knot the two ends of the cord and cut
  off the extra. The final length is up to you.

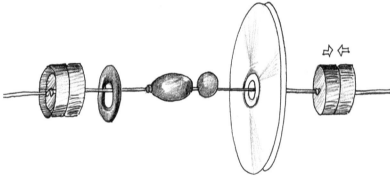

Tip: Think about arranging the objects to provide surprises and
discovery. For instance, you can place the caps in such a way
that when close together (open surfaces facing each other)
they hide a third smaller cap.

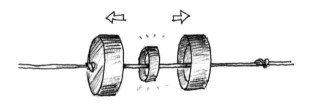

DISCOVERY TUBE

Decorate a cardboard mailing tube with self adhesive decorative paper (silver or glittery for example). You can provide the tube with inviting tactile experiences on the outside as well as putting interesting objects inside for the person to discover. The tube can also be shaken to produce various sounds, depending on the contents.

MATERIALS
cardboard mailing tube
  25cm/10″ long
fabric scraps
ribbons
self adhesive decorative
  paper

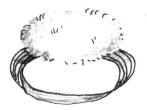

Suggestions for decorating the outside of the tube

- Make a 'bracelet' from sheepskin or other soft furry natural material and elastic. It can be slipped on and off the tube as well as worn by the person.
- Wrap a silk curtain cord around the tube and knot it loosely so it can be untied.
- Put several thick rubber bands around the tube.

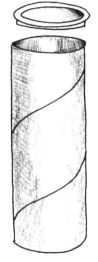

Suggestions for objects to put into the tube

- Old keys on a chain
- Small hand exercise ball
- Bag of coins
- Wooden forms sanded smooth on cord (try to avoid obvious baby toys).

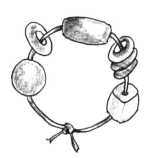

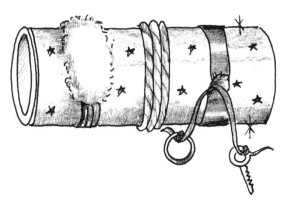

115

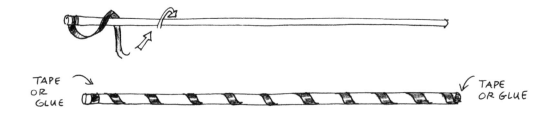

TAPE
OR
GLUE

TAPE
OR GLUE

MUSIC AND MOVEMENT WAND

1 Wrap a bamboo stick or wooden dowel with decorative tape.

MATERIALS
wooden dowel or
 bamboo stick
 30cm/12″ minimu

decorative tape

ribbons

sticky tape

glue

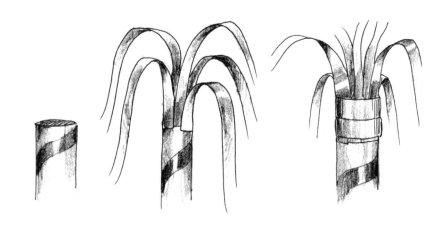

2 Fasten varicoloured ribbons to the end of the stick with tape or glue.

Use the music wand to keep time to music together; or take it outside on a windy day; or use in a group to make large, graceful arm movements with or without music.

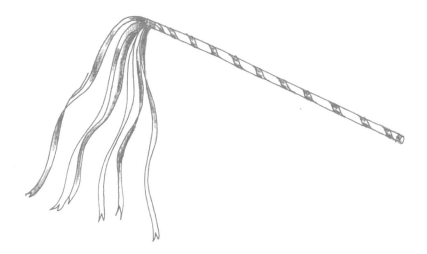

SOFT CLOTH

A cloth with an interesting print can be used to wipe the table surface, dust with, or can become a companion.

SOFT BALLS

There are a number of these available in various materials.They can be rolled over the table from person to person. Or aimed into a bucket on the floor or on the table as basketballs. Or to play 'catch' with.

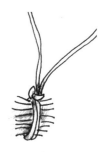

WOOLLEN POM-POM

1 Cut two rings out of cardboard (±9cm/3½" outside circle, ±3cm/1¼" inside circle).

MATERIALS
cardboard
yarn
yarn needle
scissors
(essential oil)

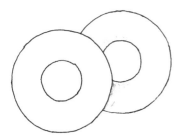
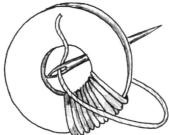

2 Thread yarn on a yarn needle and wrap around the two rings quite thickly until the centre hole is almost filled.

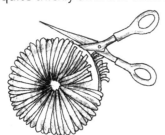
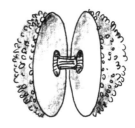

3 Insert point of scissors and cut the yarn apart along the small space between the two rings.
Thread a double length of yarn in between the two circles as shown and knot it. Gently pull the cardboard rings off (sometimes you have to cut them away).

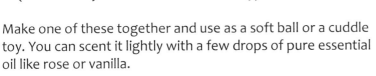

Make one of these together and use as a soft ball or a cuddle toy. You can scent it lightly with a few drops of pure essential oil like rose or vanilla.

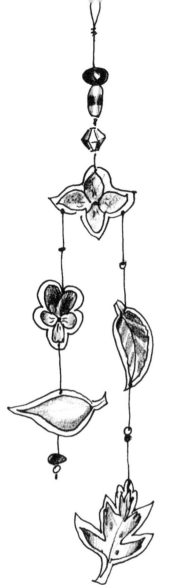

To make for the room

These are also low/no cost activities and can be done with individuals or a group, but I often do them for people who can no longer use their manual skills. The results cheer up any room and are especially suited as a quiet activity to do sitting with bedridden people. The mobiles and decorations can be hung, taped, pinned, sewn or otherwise attached to curtains, ceilings, IV poles, bulletin boards, and other surfaces.

Try to personalise these as much as possible, for example, by hanging a decorative name tag on a mobile or using the person's favourite colours, scents or photos.

HANGING FLOWER STREAMERS AND MOBILES

Using dried flowers or leaves, sandwich in between clear self-adhesive plastic and fairly heavy weight acetate (can be bought, or cut from supermarket vegetable packaging). Punch holes at the top and bottom and thread as shown to the left.

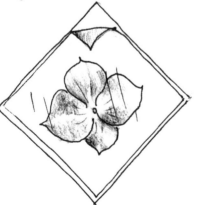
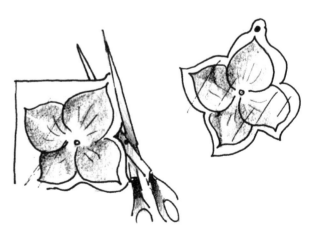

SMALL MANDALAS

Drawn circular designs or other decorations can be prepared
and hung in the same way as the flower streamers.
See *Mandalas* (p162).

POTPOURRI BAGS

To make simple potpourri bags:

1   Cut out rounds of fabric. Use pinking shears for decorative
    finished edges.

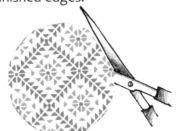
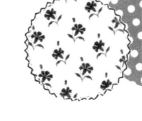

2   Sew in a long running stitch several millimeters in
    from the edge.

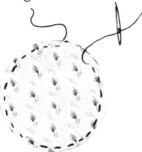

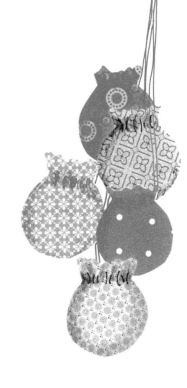

3   Gather, and fill with potpourri mix.
    These can be hung in festive, sweet-smelling bunches.

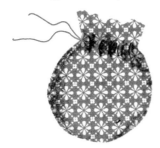

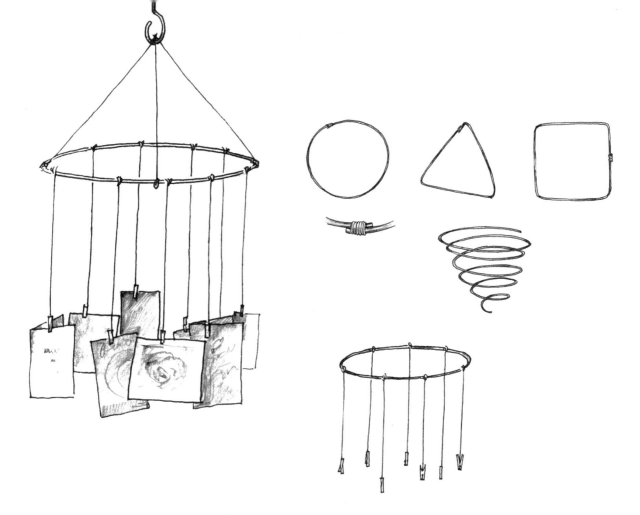

CARD MOBILE

The card mobile is a response to the fact that notice boards are so often behind people's beds, and therefore out of their sight, especially if the person is bedridden. This mobile is meant to be hung above the bed near the foot end.

Use thick wire and make a circle or other form (±24 cm/9½"). If you like, you can decorate this wire by wrapping it with coloured papers, ribbons or cord. Thread separate cords or threads on at intervals as shown (embroidery thread or decorative cord). Attach mini clothes pegs to the end of each cord, and clip cards on. If the person you are making this for doesn't receive cards, make sure they do!!

MATERIALS
thick wire
thin wire
thread or cord
paper clips or
mini clothes pegs
pliers for bending wire

'STAINED GLASS' FORMS

Use heavy black paper (or another colour if preferred) and tissue- or kite paper for the 'glass'.

MATERIALS

black or coloured paper
  120 gm or heavier
tissue or kite making
  paper in various colours
white pencil
craft knife
scissors
glue
thread for hanging

1 Fold the black paper in half and draw a pattern on it with white pencil.

2 Cut a pattern through **both** thicknesses with a craft knife.

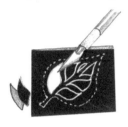 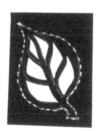

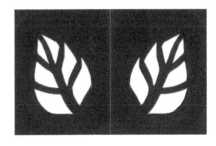

3 Open the paper out and glue one sheet of coloured transparent paper between the two layers.

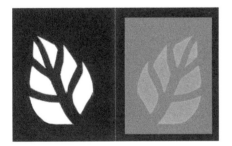 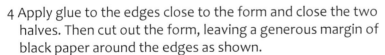

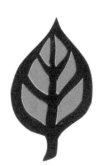

4 Apply glue to the edges close to the form and close the two halves. Then cut out the form, leaving a generous margin of black paper around the edges as shown.

Hang or stand near a lamp or window where the light will shine through the tissue paper.

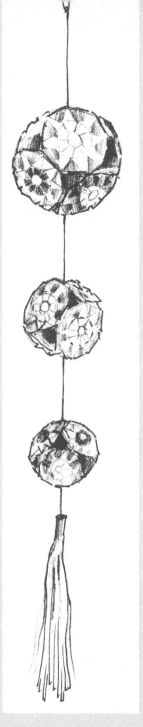

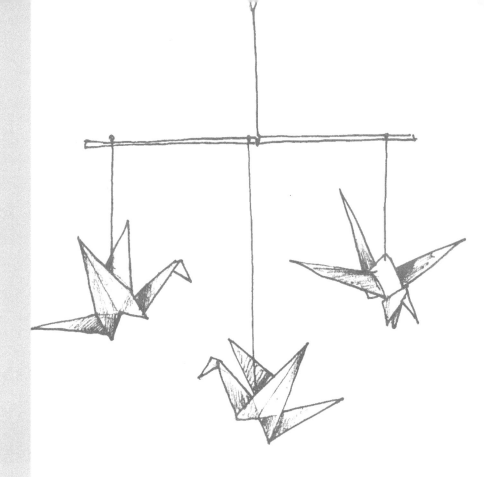

ORIGAMI BIRDS AND KUSUDAMAS
Look in a craft book or online for directions for making either origami animals or geometric forms. Make a mobile from the finished pieces.

PHOTO COLLAGE
Nice to hang on the wall or notice board. Choose a theme: *A trip or vacation, In and around the house and garden, or Friends, etc.*

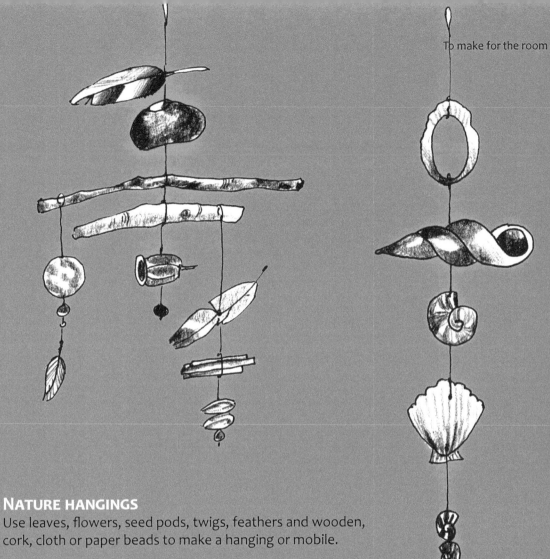

NATURE HANGINGS

Use leaves, flowers, seed pods, twigs, feathers and wooden, cork, cloth or paper beads to make a hanging or mobile.

NAME SILHOUETTE HANGERS

See *Letters and handwriting* (p144) for directions.

Paper flowers for adorning lamps, IV poles, curtains, notice boards, wheelchairs, etc.

CRINKLE FLOWER

MATERIALS

Needle or awl for punching holes

Thin wire for stem

Tissue paper in various colours

Scissors

Pencil

Needle-nosed pliers-(optional)

1 Cut 2 circles from cardboard to use as patterns, one 8cm/± 3¼" and the other 10cm/±4" in diameter.

2 Fold some light coloured tissue paper until you have 6 layers, trace the 8cm pattern onto the folded tissue and cut through all layers.

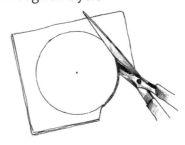

3 Repeat this with a darker coloured tissue paper and the 10 cm pattern. You now have two stacks of circles each with 6 layers of paper.

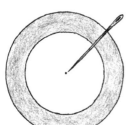

4 Centre the circles on top of each other, the smallest one on top and make a hole in the middle with a needle, pull a length of wire through (about 14 cm/5½") and coil one end with pliers so the paper circles don't fall off.

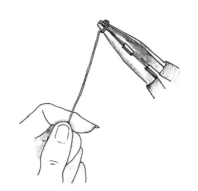
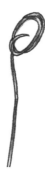
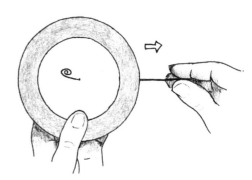

5   Coil the wire close to the back of the flower as shown to
    hold all the layers in place.

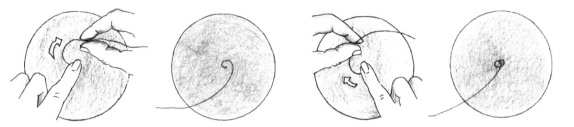

6   Turn the flower over so that the small circle is visible as
    shown and begin to crinkle the 'petals' one by one. Not too
    tightly and not too loosely. Don't worry if your flower looks
    different from the illustrated one, everyone's is different.

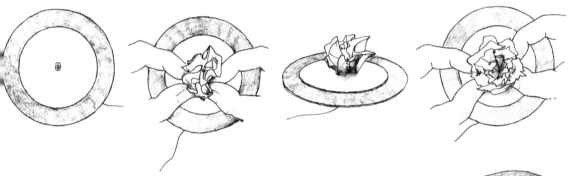

7   You will probably have to play around with the petals a bit
    to get a full looking flower. If they are too tightly scrunched,
    gently prise them apart. If they are loose and don't resemble
    a carnation, you might have to crinkle them tighter.

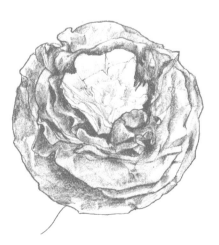

Activities based on former professions

Offering activities based on former work is an area where you might need to tread carefully. It may seem obvious to us that someone who made her living as a dressmaker would enjoy picking up a needle and thread again, but the opposite can be true. Often because of reduced abilities the person becomes frustrated when reminded of what they used to be good at. Still, you can approach this indirectly by focusing on materials and sensibilities rather than literal tasks and objects.

There was a former seamstress in my group at the home. I offered her an array of sewing materials and she responded happily to seeing them.

She didn't sew, but she did interact with the materials in her own way, for example, by repeatedly smoothing small patches of fabric in her lap.

Here are some suggestions for activities loosely linked with former areas of work:

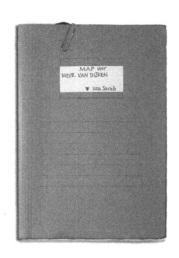

MANAGER OR OTHER AUTHORITY POSITION
Include the person on decision-making discussions, let them observe meetings if appropriate, treat with the same respect as if they still held a leadership position. If in a nursing home, find ways to give them a say in the running of their wing.
Make a clipboard for them.

SECRETARY, OFFICE ASSISTANT
Provide the person with office supplies. Is there an internal phone they could answer sometimes? Give them small tasks to do such as stuffing an envelope or pinning an announcement up on a bulletin board. See 'Office folder' next page.

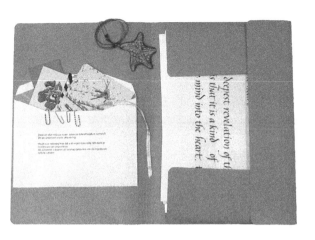

THE OFFICE FOLDER: Fill an old notebook or folder with out-of-date official papers. Add writing materials, and discovery pockets. The one I made for Mrs van D included old decorative gift tags, block print designs, paint sample cards, calligraphic practice pages, glittery cards and ribbons, stickers, and other materials I had in my studio.
Write the person's name on the front of the file, and decorate a name tag for them to wear. (Also see story p43-44.)

TEACHER
Provide chalk board and chalk and other school supplies: fresh paper, notebook, pencils, sharpener. Have the sharpener mounted and bring pencils for them to sharpen regularly.
Organize supply rooms or supply room drawers together.
See if the person shows interest in maps or textbooks. Ask for their help in performing an easy task such as punching holes in paper. Or ask their advice on something you know they know.

ELECTRICIAN, PLUMBER
Provide tools, pipes, plastic covered wires. Certain large plastic tubing can be fitted together in different ways as a game.
Give them an appliance to take apart or fix. Ask opinion about various tools or parts.
Stripping copper wires with a wire stripper or snipping them into small pieces could be satisfying. Bending wires into different shapes could yield creative results.

SEAMSTRESS

Give materials; needles, threads, scraps of cloth. Do simple projects like repairs, or sewing on buttons or making doll clothes. Or let the person play with/arrange the materials.

Make simple potpourri bags (p119):
Cut out rounds of fabric, sew in a long running stitch several millimetres in from the edge, gather, and fill with potpourri mix. Hang them near the bed, from IV poles, in a cupboard, or in a corner of the room.

ACTOR OR OTHER PERFORMER

Bring in dramatic clothes and make up – do photo sessions, give them a chance to perform. Make a celebrity board featuring the person with recent pictures of them dressed and made up.

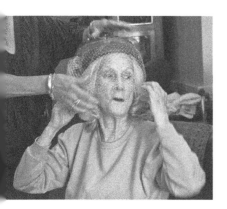

ARTIST

Provide materials and a place to work. If frustrated with old technique maybe a new medium would work – instead of painting, try sculpting or collage. Bring in pictures and art books, and catalogues and videos, and discuss or look at paintings together. Go to a museum together. Make a 'Concentration/ memory' game using pictures of famous artworks as imagery.

NURSE, DOCTOR, OTHER MEDICAL

Involve them in simple discussions about treatment, or have them hold dressings or otherwise assist in routine treatments. Let them organize a first aid box or drawer.

BUILDER, MANUAL LABOURER

Have large things for them to carry and stack. Keep them active with walking and perhaps dancing or other movement. Give them things to do with their hands involving wood, stone or clay.

LANDSCAPE DESIGNER, GARDENER

Make a miniature garden or a terrarium and have them tend it when they feel like it. Tend fish in an aquarium. Do small repotting, pruning and sowing jobs inside. Do the same in a greenhouse or outside in good weather.

Poetry writing

This chapter continues on from *Collaborative creative writing* (p96). At first it may seem contradictory to combine a skill like poetry writing with someone who has cognitive problems. But projects involving people with dementia and poetry are proven to be successful and becoming more widespread.

Using Kenneth Koch's book, *Teaching Poetry writing to Old people* as a guide, I led regular poetry writing sessions with my group. Sometimes the sessions were inspired and productive, sometimes they were less so. Determining factors on a given day could be the individual's mood, my own inspiration, and the person's willingness to try something unfamiliar.

Nevertheless, I've found that even people in more advanced stages of dementia, if patiently prompted, would speak about a subject enough for me to write down words and read them back in poetic form.

I often just started with a suggestive topic like 'my favourite colour' and asked the individuals to use the name of this colour in every line of their poem. If they had trouble thinking of a colour, I would let them choose one from different coloured papers fanned out, or objects.

One example from Mrs B:
> *Red is a good colour*
> *Red is warm*
> *I love red.*

Writing poems, people discovered things in themselves that had been hidden;

writing poems, they made these things into art.
—Koch (1997)

Imagine you are....

I am the forest,
at night I am dark
my birds sit on
branches
with their heads
tucked in their
feathers.
The moon is so high
and gold.
–Mrs G, a resident

I am the forest, and
I do have animals.
My birds fly away
sometimes, but they
also return.
I am a peaceful
place.
–Mr B, a resident

I am the forest
I'm an open wood,
where the sun shines
and all the sorrow
disappears.
–R, a student nurse

It is important to interpret the idea of 'poem' loosely. It doesn't have to rhyme or have a certain metre. Similar to *Collaborative creative writing* (p96) based on John Killick's work, I just asked the person leading questions, and built on their responses with confirming remarks or more questions, then wrote down everything they said. Next, I involved them in composing the lines by reading out what they had said and asking their agreement to my choices in line breaks.

You can work individually or write group poems. In a group, suggest a theme like 'my childhood home' and go around the circle, each person adds a phrase. Read the poem out as it grows, and read it at the end.

The ideas below come from Kenneth Koch's book, *Teaching Poetry writing to Old people* (Koch 1997).

START WITH ONE SUGGESTIVE WORD
Choose the name of a colour, for example, and repeat that in every line. Ask leading questions: 'What colour is your favourite? What does red make you think of? Did you ever have red shoes or a red hat? What was it like to wear them?'
Take cues from their answers and write down what they say.

IMAGINE YOU ARE...
For example, 'Imagine you are the ocean'. Start every line with
    'I am the ocean...
    'I am the ocean and I am running in and out...
    'I am the ocean I am huge...
    'I am the ocean full of salt...

Other suggestions for topics: *'I am the city at night'*, *forest, sky, river, desert, mountain, a stone, a tiger, a cat, a bird, a dolphin....*

BRING IN OBJECTS FOR INSPIRATION
Shells, flowers, driftwood, velvet, lace, old clothing, old utensils, gardening gloves, old packages etc. can all be suggestive. 'Tell about this object, what personal associations does it have for you'?

WRITE A COLLABORATIVE POEM IN A GROUP
Go around and invite everyone to add one phrase about the
subject – a good theme is 'these hands'. I read a poem done
this way and it was very moving, there were lines like: 'these
hands have served me well, these hands have held babies and
cleaned houses, these hands have calmed a fearful child and
caressed a loved one's face…'
Other suggestions: *My childhood home, A trip to the grocery
store when I was young, Going out on a first date…*

REFRIGERATOR POETRY MAGNETS
These are great but generally too small to handle or read easily. You could also just write groups of adjectives and nouns
on large cards. Have people pick one from each pile and from
the resulting combination, make nonsense poems. These were
wonderful opportunities for humour as in Mrs G's poem:

> *'Chocolate rain'*
>
> *Have you ever seen anything like it in your life?*
>
> *Chocolate rain,*
> *just open your mouth*
> *and swallow!*

A POETIC PORTRAIT ABOUT A LOVED ONE
Theme suggestions: *My sister, mother, husband.* If strong
feelings come up, it is fine, go with it and help the person to
express what they are feeling.

THE QUIETEST TIMES, 'THE QUIETEST THING I KNOW':
Or 'the most beautiful things I know'; 'the strangest thing that
ever happened to me'; 'I never told anybody…'; or
'My favourite things…'

Use these phrases to mine feelings and experiences.

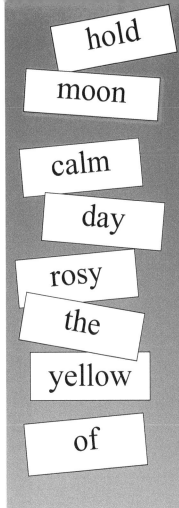

Here are some ideas on presenting the poems:

PRESENT THE POEM AS AN ARTWORK

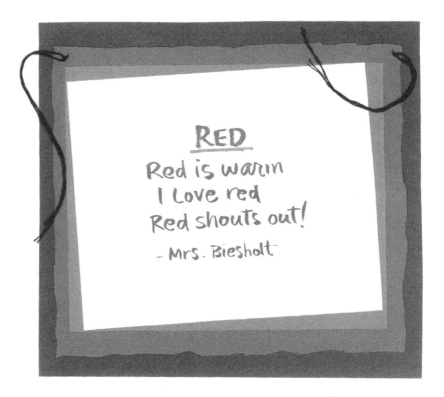

Mrs B's poem was copied out informally in brush letters, and glued onto several sheets of red, orange, and pink paper. The coloured papers' edges are roughly cut, and the white page is slightly skewed for interest.

A few red threads are sewn through more for pizazz than function. But I often do sew paper together instead of glueing, for more visual interest.

PRESENTATION BOOKLET

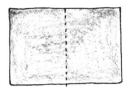 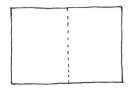 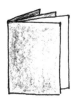

MATERIALS

1 piece of A4
(8½"x 11") 120-160g
cover paper, coloured

1 piece of A4
(8½"x 11") 80g white
or cream paper

needle and thread

1 Fold the cover and the inside sheet in half. Fit the inside into the cover. (The poem can already be written on the white sheet, check the middle illustration of the last row below for orientation.)

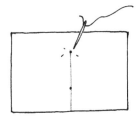 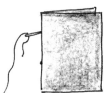 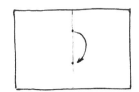 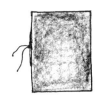

2 Thread a needle with a length of embroidery thread or other thick cotton about 25cm/10". With the needle, first punch two holes directly through all thicknesses from the inside to the outside, (don't sew yet) and hold in place. Then sew, *starting on the outside* as shown, tie a knot. Don't worry if you have done the opposite, just tie the knot on the inside.

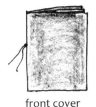 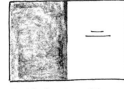 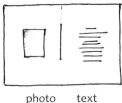 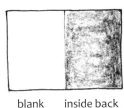 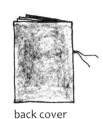

front cover   inside front   title   photo   text   blank   inside back   back cover

3 Open the front cover and write the title and author of the poem on the right hand white page. Open to the middle of the booklet and write or paste the poem inside.

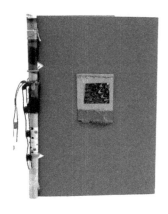

Rubber band book
see next page for directions

Making simple books

Simple books are satisfying to make; plus they are wonderful 'containers' for memories, events or themes.
Good results can be had using basic office materials, but the book turns into something of a different order when the best fine art materials are used.

The inside pages can be made from creamy rich drawing papers with torn or deckle (uncut) edges, and the covers from interesting handmade papers or heavyweight coloured drawing papers.

THEME SUGGESTIONS

A birthday gift book – a collection of snippets from friends: sketches, messages, photos etc.

New baby scrapbook – or child's first day at school etc.

Travel log – collect tickets, notes, photos, etc. from a vacation or a day trip.

Poetry – write out or print out and paste in the poetry results from one of the previous chapters. You can also collect favourite poetry from others and paste those in.

Presentation – Four page book as presentation for a poem or card or other special item. See *Poetry writing* (p133).

Memories – 'Things I'd like to remember' – either practical info or specific memories.

Collection – stamps, leaves, or photos from magazines of favourite subjects – animals, clothes, interiors, art, etc. Place in a leporello (accordion) book (p138).

RUBBER BAND BOOK

The pleasure of this easy to make book is that it can be done on the spot with normal office supplies: some printer paper, a pencil and a rubber band are all that are needed.
But, of course, good paper, a nice cover and a bamboo stick cut to size give a more sophisticated looking result.

To make the book:

1 Decorate the stick if desired.

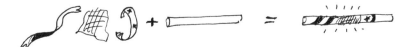

2 Fold cover.

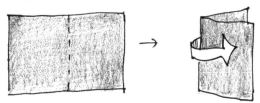

3 Fold pages and assemble as shown.

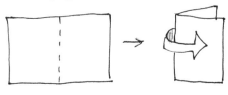 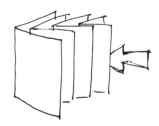

4 Center the pages in cover, cover is slightly larger.

    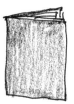 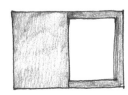

MATERIALS

A4/(8½" x 11") paper
 for pages
120-160g cover paper
pencil or bamboo
rubber band
pencil
scissors

for decorating:
 glue
 ribbons
 unusual papers
 fabric scraps
 other collage material

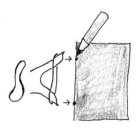

4   Lightly stretch the rubber band and mark length with pencil.

5   Make 2 V shaped cuts as shown.

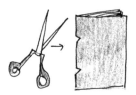   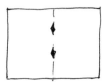

6   Open the book and stick one end of the rubber band into the upper hole (from the inside to the outside).

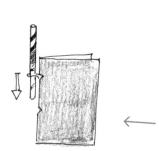

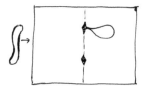   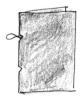

7   On the outside, slide the bottom of the bamboo stick or pencil through the rubber band loop. Don't push the whole stick through yet.

8   While holding the stick in place open the book. On the inside, stretch the rubber band and push it through the lower hole. Hold it in place once it is on the outside.

9   The next step can be fiddly: while you're keeping the rubber band stretched, close the book partially and slide the stick carefully down until you can stretch the lower loop around it. A crochet hook can be handy to catch hold of the loop while you're holding everything else.

The book is now ready to decorate!

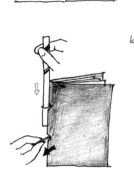

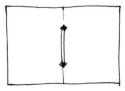   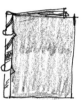

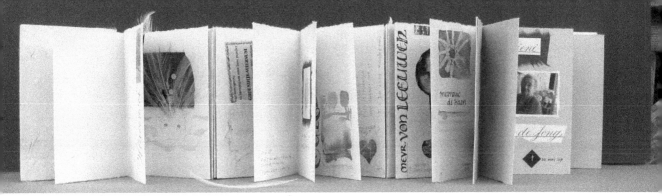

Books for you

I've added this section because making books is a simple creative act that can be an important and supportive personal ritual.

When I first started working as a volunteer in a psychiatric nursing home, five people on the ward died in the first half year I worked there. I felt that if I were to stay for a long time, I'd most likely witness more deaths, and I didn't want to forget even one of the unique individuals I had got to know.
So I started a personal memory book which marked the passing of each person I'd worked with. Each time someone died, I started a new page and calligraphed their name on it accompanied by drawn or collaged associations I had with that person. Sometimes on the back I wrote a personal message of thanks to them. Not only did the making of these pages serve as a factual recording of the deaths of the people I'd known at the home, but it became a deeply comforting ritual to remember each person in letters and images. It was a tribute to each one as well as a way for me to deal with their passing.

Perhaps you will find your own special purpose for a little book that you make, which will fulfil some need that you have in relation to your work or care for someone with dementia.

LEPORELLO OR ACCORDION BOOK

Begin with a long strip of paper; the length is about 5x the width. For example: 10cm x 50cm (4"x 20").

1 Fold the strip of paper in half as shown.

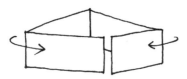 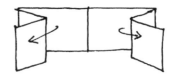

2 Fold the sides toward the middle.

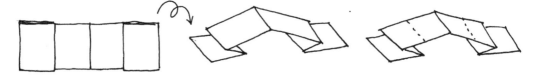

3 Now fold back the sides so the the edges are precisely even with the folds just made.

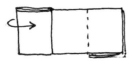 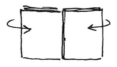 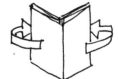

4 Turn it over, the dotted lines show where the next folds will be made.

5 Fold the left and right sides to the middle as shown. Fold in half on the middle fold.

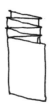 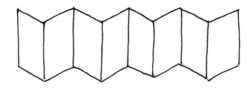

Violá, a leporello

COVERS

Use a piece of heavy coloured paper. Measure it about 5mm (¼″) larger in height than the leporello (based on the example given it will be 10,5cm, or 4¼″ high). Make two.

MATERIALS
paper 80g
cover paper 120gm
decorative papers
glue
ruler
scissors

1   Fold in half as shown.

  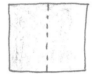

2   Close the top and bottom by glueing on any shape of patterned or contrasting paper you like. This forms one pocket cover.

3   Slip the pocket covers on either end of the leporello. You can tie a ribbon around it if you wish. The book can now be filled in any number of ways, see themes on next page.

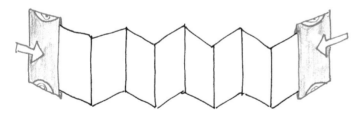

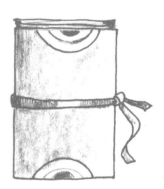

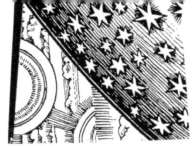

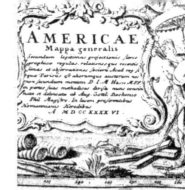

AMERICAE
Mappa generalis

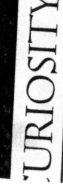

wonder...is pleasure in itself.

is the stick. ★ Togeth

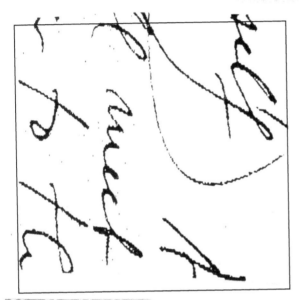

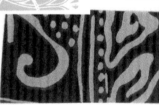

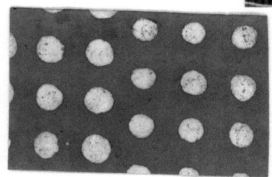

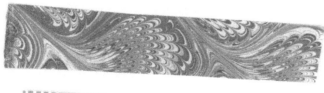

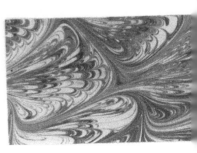

Record activity **ideas and inspirations** from this book, your own experience and elsewhere

A book for recording **special moments** with people you work with or care for

A book of interesting or **funny comments** of residents or patients

Memories or moments from the individual's past you want to keep safely for them

Your own **thoughts or poetry**

Sketches

A collection of **inspirational and consoling quotes** and ideas

Recipes of the persons's favourite foods, or family recipes you want to record before they get lost

A purely **decorative book,** made beautiful by the addition of natural materials, papers, ribbons and fabrics

A book like the one described on p137 – **'In memory of'.**

THEME SUGGESTIONS

Left-hand page: When saving decorative papers to glue in books or on the pocket covers for the leporello described on the previous pages, don't overlook scraps of interesting handwriting, copies of old engravings, and bits of type.

Letters and handwriting

I am including this chapter because my own background as a calligrapher led to a several activities where letters played an important part.

You don't have know how to do calligraphy to have fun with letters. I found that even if someone is having trouble reading, they can often recognize their name, or just the shapes of separate letters.

Writing and writing-like movements often stay imprinted even in cases of severe memory loss. The ideas in this chapter can be done for or with someone; for more complicated projects you can begin the activity, and proceed by giving a different task to each person. For example, one person could cut out what you've drawn, someone else can paste.

NAME CARDS

Using markers or any other writing tool that is comfortable for you, write the person's name large on a piece of coloured card or a tag. You can frame it as suggested in the section on collage and tape or tack it to the door. These can also be decorative additions to walking frames.

ABCDEFGH
IJKLMN
OPQRST
UVWXYZ

1234567890 &!

abcdefghijk
lmnopqrstu
vwxyz

MATERIALS

light card or heavy
 paper (10cm x 29cm/
 ±4″ x 11½″) –
 1 sheet of white and
 1 sheet of a dark colour
 or black

craft knife

scissors

thread and needle

optional – beads

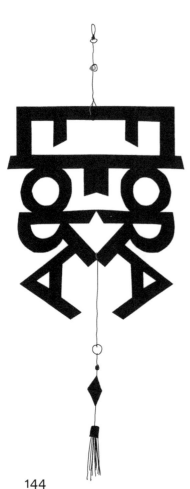

NAME SILHOUETTE HANGER

1 Draw the letters of the person's name on a piece of heavy white paper – it will fit on 1/2 of an A4/(8½″ x 11″) lengthwise. You can use the alphabet shown on p143 or find lettering styles in calligraphy books, typeface sample books or on the internet.
Compose the name so that all the letters touch.

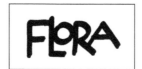 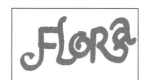

Tip: Try varying the size of the letters, combining capitals and small letters in the name, or adding a few curls.

2 Cut out the name *all in one piece*, using a knife to cut the inner shapes, like the ones in the 'O' and 'R'.

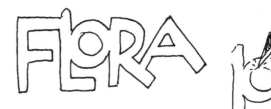

3 Fold a piece of black or dark coloured A4 paper in half lengthwise.

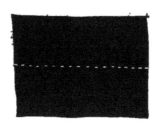 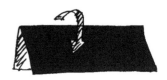

4 Place the cut-out with the *bottom of the letters on the* **fold**
   and trace around them with a light-coloured pencil.

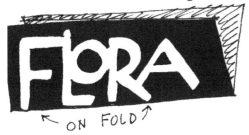
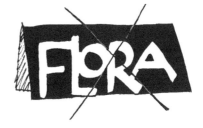

5 Keep the paper folded and cut as in step 2. Be sure to cut
   through both layers.

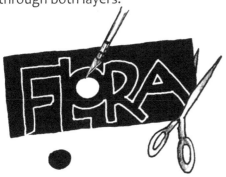
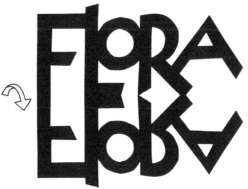

6 Open the paper out and you see the name in silhouette, one
   half is a mirror image.

   Thread a string through the top and hang in a window
   or on a wall.
   You can add other decorations such as beads or cut-out
   paper shapes or fringes.

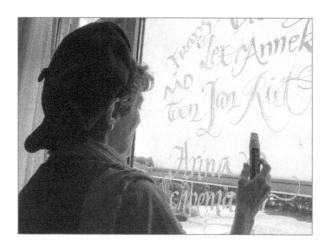

WINDOW DECORATION

Buy a broad tipped window marker and write the person's name on the window of their room.

Using decorative scripts, you can write the names of the children and grandchildren too. These markers are easy to wipe off with a dry or wet cloth unless you leave them on for more than a few weeks.

HANDWRITING

If the person likes to use a pen or felt tip, provide a large sheet of paper and demonstrate how to create all kinds of loopy, swirling letters. They can be legible or not and only loosely related to letters. These sheets can be used as raw material for further colouring in, to make cards, collages, or wrapping papers.

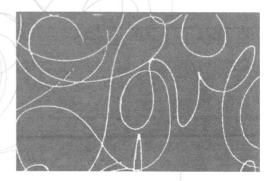

ALPHABET DESIGNS

Write a capital alphabet placing the letters in pleasing positions to form a composition. Try varying this by making the letters different sizes. These can be coloured in later.

CUT-OUT ALPHABET

The alphabet below was cut directly out of card with scissors. I didn't draw it beforehand, but each letter can be drawn first if you like. Use one or more colours for the alphabet and paste the letters on a contrasting background. I glued them down and arranged them as I went, but you can also cut first and arrange all the letters before gluing.

the dotted line shows where I went in to cut out the inside of the A

With the inside of the D I did the same – once glued down the cut disappears

You can even skip cutting out the inside of the letter – see the P

The tilt of the L was suggested by the form of the K.

ABCD EFGHIJKL MOPQRST NU VWXYZ

Letters tilting, variations in size and thickness all make this alphabet bold and playful. SZ

147

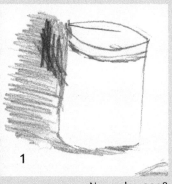

1

November 2008

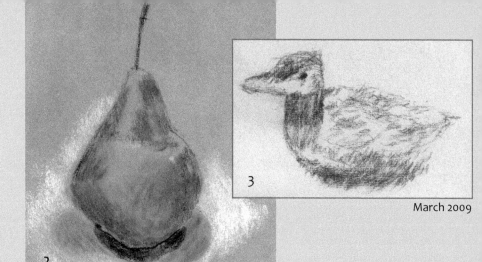

2

December 2008

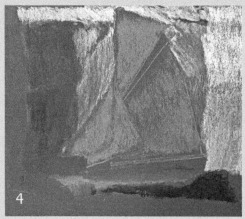

3

March 2009

These drawings were made by a friend of ours who attended weekly private drawing lessons with me for a year and a half.

He had suffered some brain damage and sketching was one of the few activities that held his interest.

The cup was his first drawing and numbers 2 & 3 show his progress over the next months.

From the end of 2009 to the beginning of 2010, he suffered severe cognitive losses. He lost the ability to translate what he saw onto the page. So I drew outlines for him to fill in (number 4).

His last drawing, number 5, was of a still life, but is no longer recognisable as such. However he worked for an hour and clearly gained pleasure from the repetitive and gentle strokes of the soft pencil.

The result is not a 'failed' attempt at drawing, but can be judged on its own merit as a sensitive abstract with lovely tone and texture.

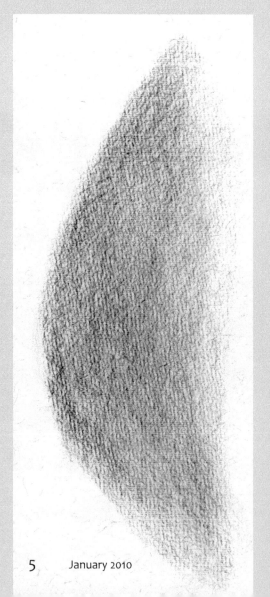

4

December 2009

5   January 2010

Drawing as visual communication

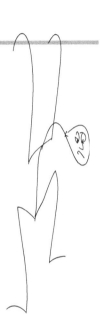

Drawing is a skill that can be learned, but even in the beginning stick figure stage, it can be a powerful communication tool.

Even if you are not a champion artist/draftsman, you can still draw at a basic level. Anyone can spontaneously sketch the floor plan of a room or the route to the supermarket; when we unself-consciously use drawing to explain something, we can do it, because no one (including our inner critic) is judging whether it is art or not! There are no 'bad' drawings when using a line as a means of communication.

You don't have to draw well, in fact awkward-looking drawings often result in fits of laughter and offers to help. See *The charm of imperfect drawings* (p154).

The ideas in this section are especially interactive, in that you start out the activity and invite the person to participate.

G, the dear lady who made the paper doll pictured on the next page, was accomplished in crafts but insisted she couldn't draw.

Facing a blank page can be intimidating. To make it easier for her to begin, we used a mini whiteboard for easy correction. (See page 65 for how to make one.)

I started by drawing part of an oval for the face and invited G to fill in the features. Gradually, as we laughed with each addition, she became more confident and added curly hair, then a neck, arms, legs and a torso. I refrained from commenting on the content or proportions, I only suggested additions.

I took the whiteboard to the copy machine and made several copies of the figure. I pasted one on white cardboard and cut it out; then we set about clothing 'Samy'.

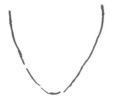

This is the basic shape I drew for G to start with.

As this woman became easily overwhelmed when she had to take the initiative, I suggested which piece of clothing we could work on next, like an earring or a blouse. We looked through magazines for the right colours and textures to clothe the doll with. It was a riot from beginning to end. I just love this expressive figure she made. This activity led to sequels: new clothes for Samy's wardrobe, the creation of a male companion, and stories about the two of them.

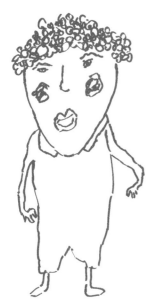

'Samy' without makeup, earrings or clothes

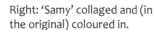

Right: 'Samy' collaged and (in the original) coloured in.

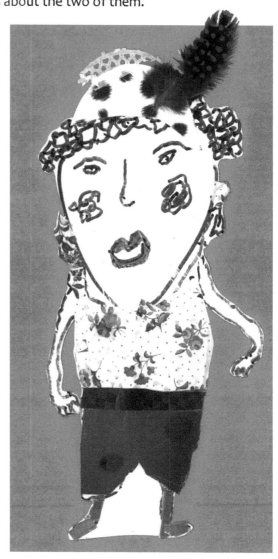

FACES

This is a simple exercise that can lead to unexpected kinds of engagement.

Simply draw an oval as shown in the illustration and ask some-one to fill in one feature, say the eyes or nose or mouth. The shape of your initial oval will influence the other features. Take turns drawing features (each new added feature is shown in black). If the person becomes more interested you can go on to hair and even a body and clothes. (See *Paper dolls* below).

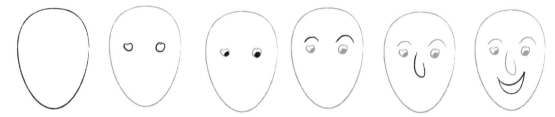

FACES AND EMOTIONS

A variation on *Faces* is to draw the oval, then ask the person to draw in a certain expression, like 'anger', or 'happiness'. You can go through a whole range of emotions this way. Or you can draw the expressions and begin a discussion based on one of them. For example, 'How do you think this person feels?' You could mimic the expression and invite the person to join you. Note: the purpose of this activity is engagement and fun, so keep the tone light.

Try out different sizes of ovals, one person may be comfortable drawing on a face that covers a whole page, someone else might prefer working on the size shown here.

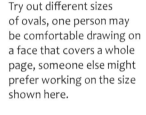

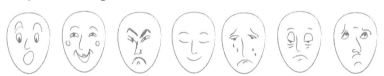

PAPER DOLLS

Follow the procedure described in the introduction for making a doll like Samy. This doesn't have to be a girl thing, for men you could make character-types like a politician, farmer, sales-man, movie star. And you could give these characters acces-sories to fit with the role. You can paste the clothes on or leave them loose as you wish.

For more ideas see, *Creative thinking* (p58).

'I live with my mother and father, my brother still lives at home, my younger brother Jipp.

It's an old fashioned house next to the quarry, and it had sleeping cubbies.

The dining room adjoined the kitchen. The kitchen had a big coal oven with rings ontop for cooking, and a cover.

Mother stoked the coal oven first thing in the morning and tended it all day.
The kitchen was warm and cozy, we all liked to sit there...'

—memories of Mrs B

HOUSES, GARDENS, AND NEIGHBOURHOODS

Contrary to what I've heard about avoiding talking about people's losses, I found that many individuals wanted to tell me about the homes they had lived in. Even though these were occasionally sad discussions, I felt that asking about their home was a way to affirm that they once had had one and relive what it was like. If it seemed appropriate, we would draw a floor plan together.

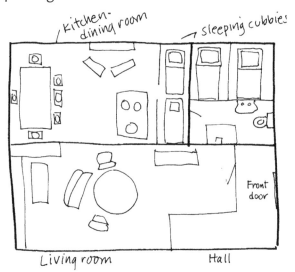

This activity is also fun to do when people are reminiscing about their *childhood* homes: 'Where was the bathroom, where did your parents sleep, where did the kids sleep? The dog, etc?' Use pencil and paper and make a floor plan of each storey of the house.

Gardens

You can draw or collage a garden for someone who misses theirs. If you feel comfortable drawing flowers, trees, etc, you can do so. But you could also collect some gardening magazines and create a garden with collaged elements.

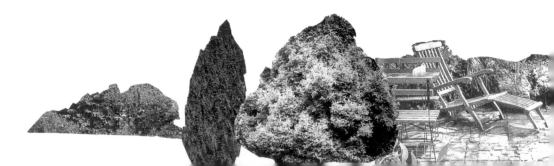

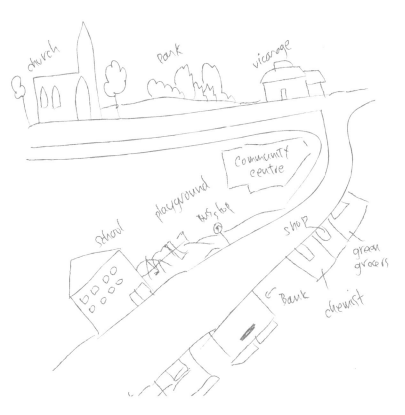

Villages and neighbourhoods

Use questions, prompts and examples to make a map of the person's old neighbourhood. Where was the church, the grocers, the dairy, etc? Let the activity grow naturally, maybe they or you want to draw buildings or other landscape features on a separate paper and paste these onto the map. The maps can become themes for other reminiscing activities, like school, friendships, first jobs, paper rounds, etc.

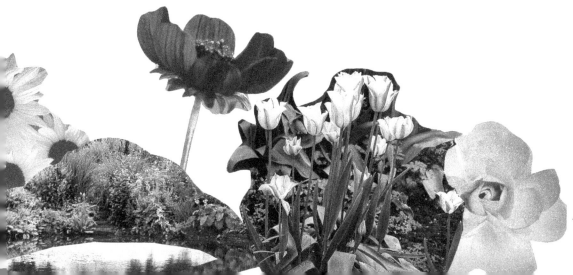

153

THE CHARM OF 'IMPERFECT' DRAWINGS

If you really can't draw, this can be turned into an advantage. Agree to draw something for the person, their home or village, a situation, or a dream they would still like to have fulfilled; and make a joke out of not being able to draw well. Make the silliest drawing you can and laugh together, you might even invite the person to try and do a better one. Working on it together can lead to surprising results.

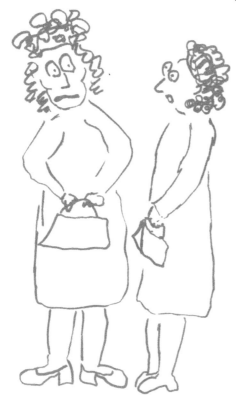

The delightful drawings on this page were made by our friend, Candy, teacher of creative writing. It is very clear that a shocking piece of gossip or other juicy information has been conveyed to the lady on the left.

You see that one doesn't have to get the arms, hands or faces 'right' to express an encounter or an emotion.

In fact, this drawing is as good as many professional cartoonists' work who also rely more on expression of line than perfect representation to communicate a message.

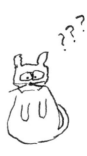

DOCUMENTING YOUR/THEIR WORLD

Simple drawings are a way of documenting your/their world;
inspired by Keri Smith's books and web site (see p183),
try one of these ideas for or with someone:

- Document everything the person ate today with a
  simple line drawing; if the person doesn't remember,
  draw an imaginary meal.

- Draw all the different kinds of chairs in the home.

- Draw the clothes you are wearing as if they were on a
  washing line.

- Draw a favourite pet from the past or present.

- Draw your favourite... tool, (book, piece of clothing,
  jewellery, car, bike).

- Take the person, in memory, back to their home and in the
  imagination go to their bedroom or kitchen or workplace.
  Now imagine a catchall drawer, and name the contents one
  by one. Below is a re-creation of this exercise done with a
  bedroom drawer. The woman did not volunteer information but was interested in the game, so I gave prompts to
  which she clearly said yes or no. 'Did you keep perfume in
  this drawer? There are usually one or two combs or hair-
  grips, what about face powder? A children's toy? Did you
  keep old love letters in there? No? well let's put a few in
  anyway' (laughter)

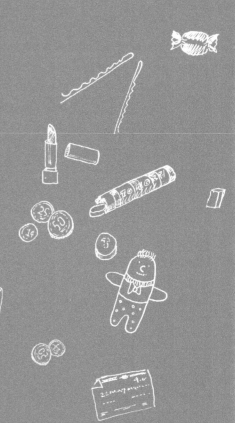
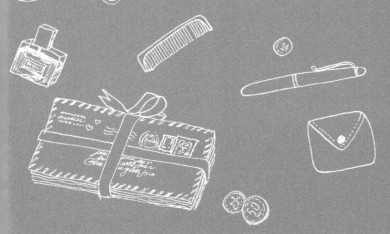

Collage

Anyone leafing through a stack of old magazines will see that many of them are luxury objects. Printed on heavy, glossy paper, they contain excellent photographs, art and design, decorative patterns, and letters. These elements can be used individually or in combination to create refreshingly aesthetic collage projects. The addition of other papers and materials can enhance the collages further, and if you add 3-D objects, it becomes an assemblage.

THE SIMPLEST COLLAGE
Leaf through magazines together and cut out the first picture the person responds to. 'Frame' it on a piece of heavy card (white or coloured) and decorate if you wish:
  a. Stick thin ribbons around the edge as a frame.
  b. Marker or coloured pencil border.
  c. Add on wrapping paper or other paper decoration.
  d. Cut a border from the same or another image from the magazine as shown below.

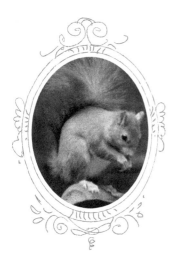

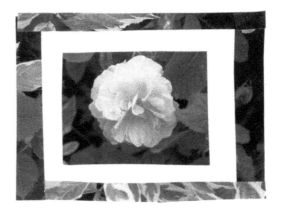

HUMOROUS COLLAGE
Cut out different objects and arrange them in absurd or surprising ways, for example: a big shoe with a tiny child inside it, a dog with a city on its back, a duck in evening clothes, etc.

COLLAGE ON A THEME
Search for images based on a specific theme such as: *vacation, gardens, cars, buildings, etc.* Cut out everything you can find even loosely related to the theme and arrange and glue on a page. Don't forget letters and words, these may be used as a title or may form part of the overall design.

GROUP COLLAGE
With around six people at a table, collage on a theme (see above). Let everyone contribute to the cutting and pasting according to what they can do. If there are more than six people, have at least two helpers for the project.

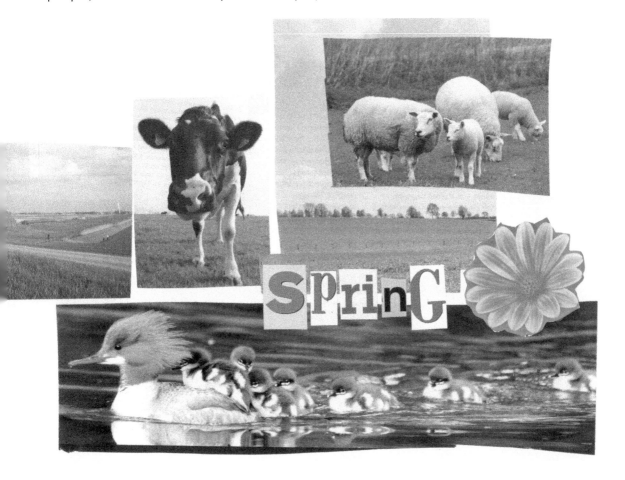

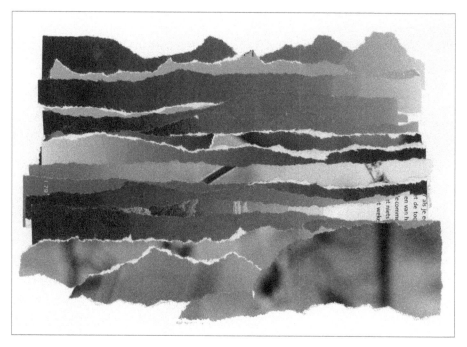

elegant
SUITS TO
Enhance
All
THE COWBOYS

CUT AND TORN
Try only tearing out shapes or combine torn and cut edges for an interesting effect.

WORD JAZZ
Search for words to make poems or nonsense sentences. Big type can be used for emphasis. All kinds of different sizes and styles make it more interesting.

Why trust just anyone with your favorite fairy godmother ?

ABSTRACT COLLAGES

These don't portray concrete subjects like a face or a flower, instead they are based on visual art principles. The results will look more like art and be associated with feelings rather than a specific subject.

For example, roughly tearing jagged shapes will convey a different feeling from a carefully cut-out collage.

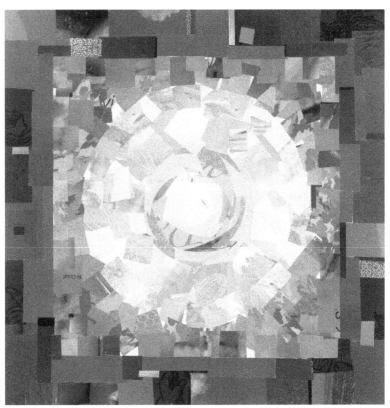

Make a collage out of big torn shapes placed randomly on the page.

Make a collage using small, carefully cut out or torn shapes and arrange into a design.

Make a blue collage by cutting out shapes wherever you find a blue area. For example: sky, water, walls in shadow, letters, furniture, clothing, etc. This is based on the visual principles of harmony and unity.

Make a blue (or any other colour) collage and add one accent of another contrasting colour. For blue it would be orange or red, for example.

Gradating is more complex but gives pleasing results: make a collage where the colour gradually changes from light to dark. See photo this page.

TISSUE PAPER COLLAGE

This technique is exciting because it is transparent and the glue or medium makes the colours run, creating surprising effects. Use a white cardboard background.

a. Use white glue slightly diluted if you like, or acrylic medium (either gloss or matte will work). Pour this out in a small dish so you can brush it on.

b. Cut or tear shapes out of various colours of tissue paper, light ones show transparency well.

c. Brush the glue onto the background (applying wet media directly onto the tissue paper makes it difficult to handle) and place the shapes on it, brush more glue over the shape, overlap shapes for transparent effects.

I've added dried flowers to the example shown. The main colours are purples, hot pinks and oranges, with some green accents. With this technique, wrinkles and tears add to the visual interest.

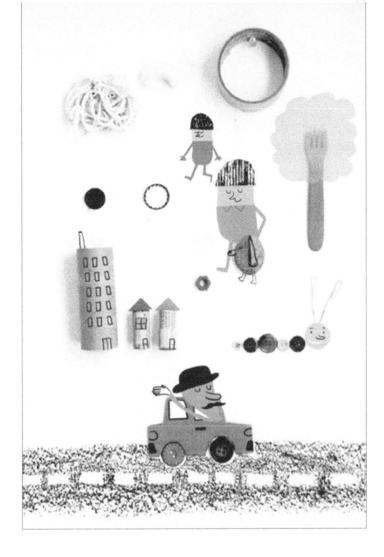

SUGGESTED MATERIALS
Pictures from
 magazines
Old family photographs
Feathers
Stick-on 'jewels'
Wrapping paper
Rice paper
Fabric scraps
Tissue paper
String
Buttons

Found City
by Keri Smith

ASSEMBLAGE

You can make an assemblage (3 dimensional collage) on a piece of heavy card or cardboard, or you could find or make a small shallow box. Choose a theme, for example: *nest, house, mystery box, pets, my heart, my past, my children*. These boxes are wonderful vehicles for telling stories. They can also house collections of shells, feathers, seed pods, coins, and other small objects.

Line the box with paper or fabric and glue in miniatures and other materials to make an artwork.

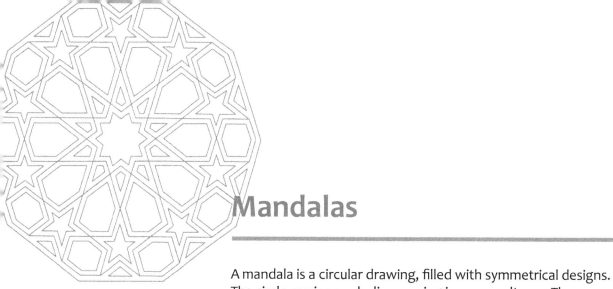

Mandalas

A mandala is a circular drawing, filled with symmetrical designs. The circle carries symbolic meaning in many cultures. The Tibetans use it as a base for intricate sand paintings which have a religious significance. The circle occurs in other religions as a symbol for the earth, sun, or cosmos.

MATERIALS
Mandala print
Coloured pencils,
  watercolour pencils,
  or felt pens

Colouring in mandalas can be a restful and rewarding activity for people with dementia. I worked on a continual basis with a woman in the middle stages of the disease who gained immense satisfaction from the beautiful drawings she completed. I worked closely with her to choose the colours most pleasing to her, and she asked my advice about certain combinations. But aside from occasional help with practical aspects, she worked independently.

You can find mandalas to colour in on the internet and in books. I've included some of G's favourite ones here. You can also create your own designs.

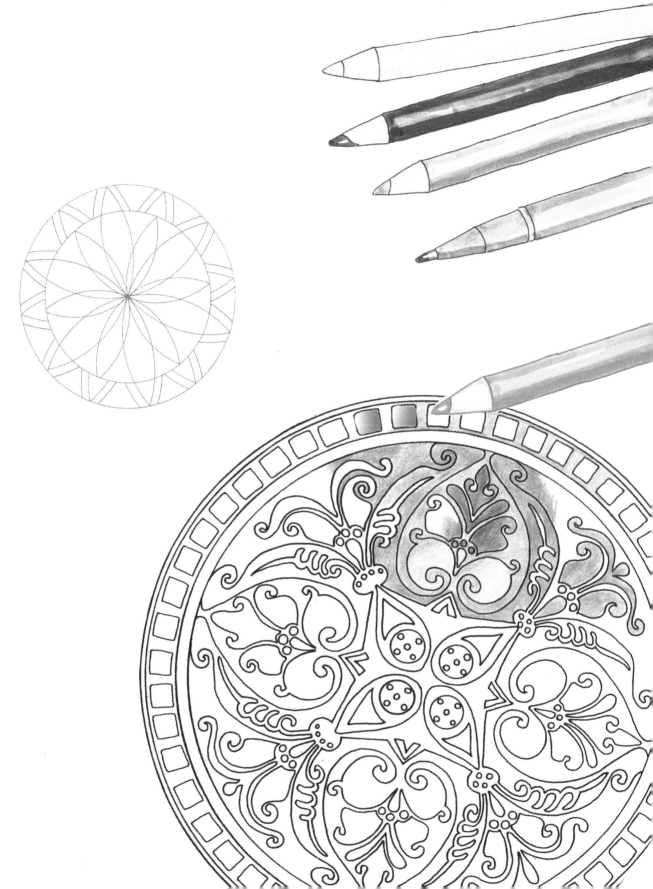

Holding

In the chapter, *Holding and physical objects* (p101), the concept of free exploration and manipulation of material as an end in itself was introduced.

To further this type of engagement you can provide a variety of materials to hold, wrap, cover, hide, pick up, examine, taste, and explore. Even the room can be a subject for interaction such as pushing against walls, or pulling at closed doors. These actions can be considered valid activities, as can becoming absorbed in the process of arranging and playing with objects in a way which indicates that this has meaning for the person.

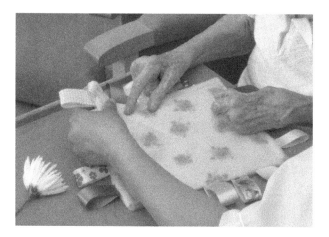

Here is a list of materials to explore and arrange:

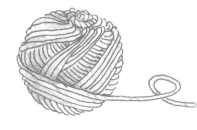

Different kinds of papers and foils
Clothes and cloth scraps
Containers with and without lids to put things into
String, rope, and balls of wool
Tape
Pencils
Rulers
Balsa wood – a soft material that can be
  easily dented, gouged or split
Stones
Sponges
Dowels
Wooden blocks or other forms
Bubble pack

Large rubber exercise balls to roll or lie on
Silverware
Doll's tea set
Miniature furniture
Doll's clothes
Contents of a hobby drawer
A collection of different sized and coloured
  balls, (tennis, ping-pong, rubber)

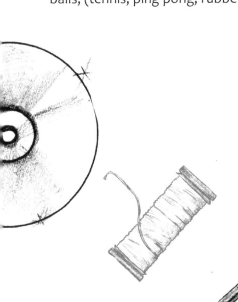

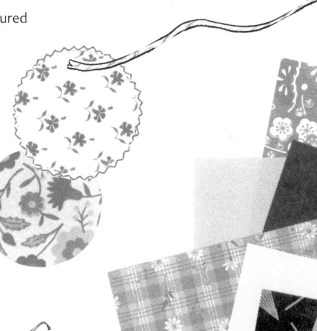

Activities based on gestures

There was a woman on my ward who, using her feet on the floor for traction, emphatically pushed herself backwards in her wheelchair. She would roll away until she encountered an obstacle, then, stuck, she began to scream until someone freed her and she could begin the whole process again.

I used to give the nursing staff a rest by taking this woman for a wheelchair stroll down the long corridors. But I didn't push the chair, I turned her around so she was facing me, I would give her a gentle shove and she would push herself backwards all the way down the hall. She enjoyed it immensely and it was great exercise for her.

Arriving back in the family room, we had a game: I gave her my scarf and she pushed herself away from me, then I would reel her in with the scarf. We did this for long periods, it was hypnotic, back then forward, back then forward, and she would become quite calm doing it.

On the following pages are other simple ways to use someone's gestures as starting points for engagement. You can use them to provide companionship and set small easily achieved tasks. (See *Start where they are* p104.)

TAPPING, PATTING

- Make a rhythmic noise together on the table using a stick or spoon, see if you can follow each other's rhythms and vary them. Go slow, fast, syncopated, three times fast, three times slow, etc.
- Pat a piece of bread dough or clay until it is flat

STROKING

- Massage someone's hands with scented cream or oil, give them a chance to reciprocate if they want
- Pet a stuffed animal
- Pet a dog, cat, rabbit or other animal
- Smooth a cloth on a flat surface or lap
- Iron a dishtowel or handkerchief (on a low setting)
- Move large wooden beads back and forth on a wooden dowel or rope
- Dry dishes

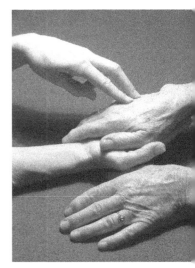

PRESSING

- Press glued paper down so it stays in place (while making a collage)
- Stamp with block print or a rubber stamp
- Press clay into a mould
- Press aluminium foil into a bowl or mould
- Make hand prints on paper or in sand or dirt
- Press the flat of your hand to theirs gently, giving and resisting in turn, taking your cues from them
- Pop the bubbles in plastic bubble pack

PULLING

- Pull the wrapping paper off a package
- Pull clothes off a doll
- Pull on a thick cord with knots
- Pull someone in a wheelchair (see story opposite)
- Hold hands gently, push and pull

OPEN PALM
- Put something edible in the centre of the palm
- Stroke or massage the palm
- Hold hands
- Draw a face in the middle of the palm with non-toxic water soluble marker
- Cover one hand with a cloth so it is hidden, pretend to find it

GRABBING, GRASPING
- Throw soft hollow-fill ball or ball of wool as a catch game
- Squeeze clay
- Scrunch paper (see *Crinkle flowers* p124)
- Play hand games where they have to catch your hand before you turn it over, or they have to grab an object covered by your hand

FOLDING
- Dish towels, clothes, bed linens
- Paper, newspaper
- Clay or dough

PICKING AT
- Peeling paper
- A torn out hem, little threads
- Make a yarn card with easy knots to untie or things to pull through loops
- Peeling a tangerine and picking away the white membranes

RUBBING
- Polish metal or shoes
- Clean stains off a surface
- Rub soft ball between hands
- Wash clothes
- Polish mirror or windows

ROLLING
- Roll clay or dough into a long snake shape
- Roll rubber tube or dowels on a table
- Roll balls on a table
- Spin wool
- Roll a cardboard tube filled with beads (securely sealed at both ends!) on a flat surface

WINDING
- Decorate a dowel by winding with string or yarn or ribbon
- Kite flying, wind reel
- Fishing, wind reel, or indoor fishing: big plastic hook, nice prizes to hook
- Decorate cardboard mailing tube with paper or yarn

WRAPPING CONCEALING
- Dressing a doll or stuffed animal
- Wrap object (box, bottle, etc.) in cloth and string
- Wrap a present
- Wrap a bandage

TEARING
- Paper strips (can be later used for papier mache)
- Cloth strips (can be used for fabric mache or other crafts)
- Tearing unneeded documents
- Tearing paper into squares for collage

WAVING/SWAYING
- Wave with *music and movement wand* (see directions for making, p116)
- Sway to music
- Wave a silk scarf to music

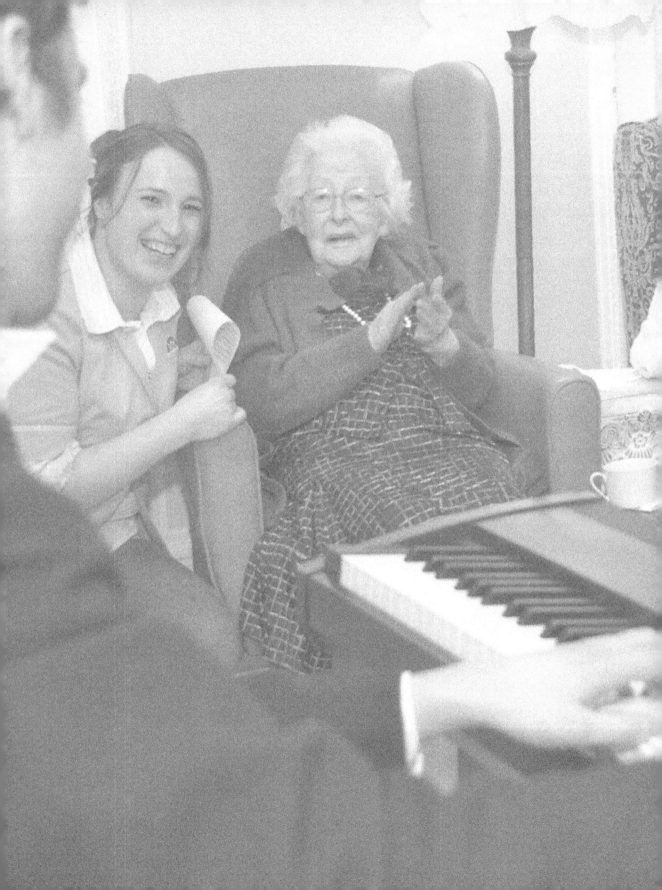

5

CLOSING THOUGHTS

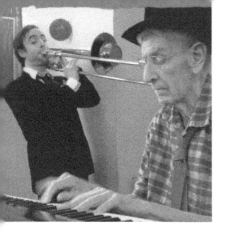

Art in dementia care

. . . .

Communication is a key concept in improving life for people with dementia, and many persons with the condition experience serious problems with language. By providing a number of alternative means of expression (mostly non-verbal) the arts may be offering the pathways they desperately need.
Killick J, Allan K (2000)

Being a visual artist, I've primarily referred to image making and working with materials in this book. There are not a lot of examples of art made by people with dementia included because I focus primarily on creativity as a catalyst for moments of encounter rather than end products.

Also, this book emphasizes that skills learned from the creative disciplines offer 'pathways' not only to people with dementia, but also to the people who care for them. Non-verbal communication, humour, the ability to take emotional risks, to improvise in the moment, etc, are not 'extras' in the field of dementia care, I consider them to be essentials.

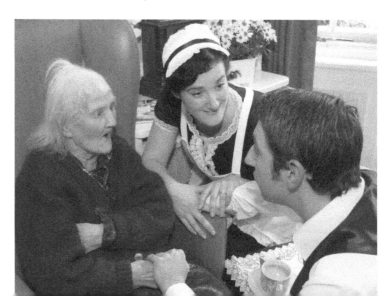

Other creative disciplines like music, dance, drama, storytelling and poetry are being successfully applied in dementia care*. The success of these types of activities lies very much with the person leading the activity. Their experience, and attitude of respect and enabling is what can turn the activity into a powerful encounter and pave the way for 'special moments'. There can be breakthroughs, such as a meeting of hearts between two people or moments of lucidity.
Though the effects can't be measured, they *can* be observed and experienced and most recent evaluations report lasting positive effects.

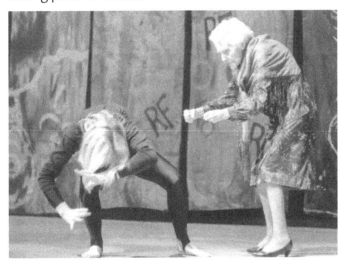

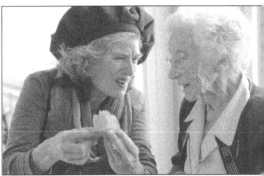

People often ask if what I do is art therapy. Though these activities may at first resemble art therapy, it is important to distinguish between an art activity and art therapy:
Art therapy uses diagnosis and planned intervention to cure or lighten symptoms.
Art activity uses creative skills to generate a sense of enjoyment, satisfaction and companionship through a moment of engagement without trying to change the person or condition.

Though the aim of art activities is not therapy, they work in a lightly therapeutic way. They can provide emotional relief, build skills and self esteem, and open avenues for expression. They may result in moments of intense interpersonal contact and lucidity.

*The Journal of Dementia Care magazine in the UK is an excellent resource for programmes and projects of this kind.

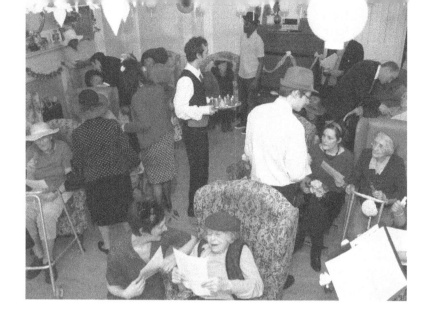

..we firmly believe that the arts in dementia care are here to stay, and not just as fringe activities but as a core component of any package of measures put together to offer positive opportunities to the individual.
—Killick J, Allan K (2000)

I am excited that the arts are gradually filtering into the health care system, and that more creative disciplines are being included in medical trainings. Some medical schools in the US offer art classes as part of the curriculum, and I heard of a programme where medical students spent time at an art museum observing paintings in order to learn subjective observation as an aid to diagnosing illness. 'After an hour at the museum, the class walked back to Harvard Medical School to apply what they had learned about examining art to diagnosing breathing problems, skin rashes, and neurological disorders, and to reading lung X-rays'. Kowalczyk L (2008).

Additionally, health institutions are inviting in qualified artists to teach creative process to staff; this is an excellent resource for inspiring health professionals to discover and use their creative abilities. The health facility gains from an infusion of creative spirit which can set off a chain reaction of positive change in the facility's culture. And artists, used to working alone in their studios, can profit from being recognised and active in a social context as well as generating a new income stream.

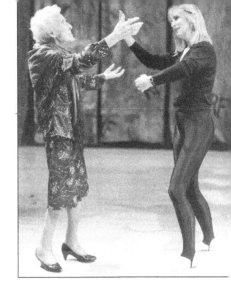

I work with a nonprofit organisation here in Holland, Beter Ge-zelschap, (loosely translated as Get Better Association) which organises large creative events in hospitals and nursing homes.

At first glance, it seems that the dancers, singers, story-tellers, artists, and actors are entertainers; but during the intense one to one contacts that occur during these days it is quickly evident that something more profound is happening. The creative disciplines are obviously bringing much needed colour, warmth, spontaneity, and a little bit of healthy chaos into the hyper technical medical environments, yet they also remind us of our shared humanity. Roles and protocols fall away leaving just human beings caught up together in a moment of wonder and connection.

I hope that reading and working with this book will add to the understanding that the arts are not distant from everyday life, but a natural and vital part of it. And that we can draw on our heart's wisdom just as much as our intellect's, to communicate and create with the people in our care.

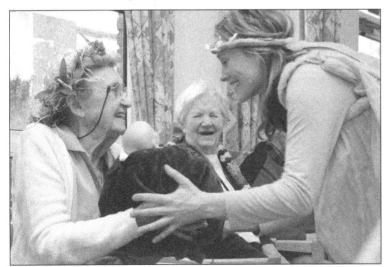

Photos in this section:
p173 left, Diane Amans/Joel Fildes
p173 right, staff photographer Care Centre
  Vroenhof, NL
This page top, Diane Amans/Joel Fildes
p170-175 all other images
  Ladder to the Moon.

MINI-GUIDES

The following is a cross-referenced source of activities grouped according to specific needs and purposes.

GROUP ACTIVITIES

Suited for, but not limited to groups

PHYSICALLY ACTIVE

QUIET, RESTFUL

Choose activities from the following chapters:

VISUAL ART

Choose activities from the following chapters:

WRITING

Choose activities from the following chapters:

Can be done one to one or with a few people

FOR A PERSON WHO CAN READ AND SPEAK COHERENTLY

Choose activities from the following chapters:

FOR A PERSON WHO CAN SPEAK BUT CANNOT READ

Choose activities from the following chapters and read the chapter on Activity grading:

Adapt the following activities to an appropriate level for the individual's abilities:

TROUBLE WITH READING, SPEAKING AND UNDERSTANDING SPEECH

Choose activities from the following chapters and read the chapter on Activity grading:

INDIVIDUAL ACTIVITIES

INDIVIDUAL ACTIVITIES *continued*

TROUBLE WITH READING, SPEAKING AND UNDERSTANDING SPEECH *continued*

Also see the chart, *Alternatives for planned activities p63*

BEDRIDDEN

Choose activities from the following chapters and read the chapter on Activity grading:

BEDRIDDEN AND NO LONGER SEEMS TO RESPOND TO STIMULI

Choose activities from the following chapters and read the chapter on Activity grading:

Try the following (activities in grey print not included in book):

Feeling textures, hand massage, bring in scented plants, roll bed to new environment, bring shells, stones and other natural objects to hold

REPETITIVE BEHAVIOUR

Choose activities from the following chapters:

SUITED TO MEN

(Most of the activities in this book are easy to do with women, but it was a special challenge to find activities to engage men.)

Choose activities from the following chapters:

STIMULATING YOUR OWN CREATIVITY
Don't forget to provide nourishment for your creative self.
Here are some chapters you can look through for suggestions and inspiration:

SIMPLE ACTIVITIES NEEDING FEW PROPS OR MATERIALS

Try one of these activities:

Walk
Listen to music
Hand massage

Choose activities from the following chapters:

ACTIVITIES LIST

BIBLIOGRAPHY

Books

Carnarius M (2015) *A Deeper Perspective on Alzheimer's and Other Dementias: Practical Tools with Spiritual Insights.* Findhorn Press.

Dowling JR (1995) *Keeping Busy: a Handbook of Activities for Persons with Dementia.* The Johns Hopkins University Press.

Killick J, Allan K (2001) *Communication and the Care of People with Dementia.* Open University Press, Buckingham/Philadelphia.

Killick J (1997) *You Are Words.* Hawker Publications, London.

Koch K (1997) *I never Told Anybody: Teaching Poetry Writing to Old People.* Teachers & Writers Collaborative, NY.

McNiff S (1998) *Trust the Process.* Shambhala, Boston, London.

Smith K (2008) *How to Be an Explorer of the World: Portable Art Life Museum.* The Penguin Group, USA.

Suzuki S (1973) *Zen Mind, Beginners Mind.* Weatherhill, New York, Tokyo.

Tolle E (1999) *The Power of Now.* New World Library, USA.

Zgola J (1999) *Care that Works: A Relationship Approach to Persons with Dementia.* John Hopkins University Press, Baltimore, MA.

Articles

Byers A (1995) "Beyond Marks, on working with elderly people with severe memory loss." Inscape Vol 1.

Biernacki C (2009) "I believe, therefore I care". The Journal of Dementia Care 17 (1) 14-15.

Colston-Taylor G (2001) "Words and stories, helping people to give feedback on services". Pathways 8.

Ferruci P (2005) "Survival of the kindest". Ode magazine 75.

Killick J, Allan K (2005) "The Good Sunset project: quality of life in advanced dementia". Journal of Dementia Care 13 (6) 22-24.

Killick J, Allan K (2000) "Undiminished possibility: The arts in dementia care". Journal of Dementia Care 8 (3) 16-18.

Kitwood T (1993) "Discover the person, not the disease". Journal of Dementia Care 1 (1) 16-17.

Kowalczyk L (2008) "New courses improve powers of observation". Boston Globe.

MORE RESOURCES AND LINKS

NAPA National Association for Providers of Activities for Older People, London
  napa-activities.co.uk

The Alzheimer's Society Book of Activities by Sally Knocker. Alzheimer's Society, UK, 2003.

Kate Allan and John Killick's web site: dementiapositive.co.uk

Books related to developing creativity
Cameron J (1994) *The Artists Way: A Course in Discovering and Recovering Your Creative Self.*
  Souvenir Press Ltd, UK.

McNiff S (1998) *Trust the Process.* Shambhala, Boston, London.

Smith K (2007) *Wreck this Journal.* Penguin and Putnam Inc, USA.

Websites
There are numerous sites encouraging creativity and recording the work of those just starting out as well as more established practitioners.

The following two sites centre on drawing:
> dannygregory.com
> michaelnobbs.com

You could also search under the term *sketchcrawl.*

Two inspiring sites for creativity:
> kerismith.com
> learningtoloveyoumore.com

For anyone feeling inspired to take up a new hobby, try the following search terms:
visual journaling, altered books, crafting, and collage.

Please note: The internet is a medium in constant flux, so we can't take responsibility for content or availability.

CREDITS

We are very grateful to the following organisations and individuals for the photographs in this book:

Diane Amans, dance artist, community dance practitioner and training consultant; Joel Fildes, photographer, for the photographs on pages 173 and 175.

Harry Giglio, photographer, for the portrait of his mother on page 13.

Cathy Greenblat, sociologist and photographer, for the photo on page 128.

Sip Hiemstra for the photo on page 47.

Ladder to the Moon, a UK-based training and theatre organisation which develops staff, builds community and shifts culture to improve the quality of life for older people in care, particularly those living with dementia.

Thanks are also due to:

All residents and staff of Compton Lodge and Rathmore House (Central and Cecil Housing Trust) and clients and staff at Wimbledon Guild day services, London who feature in the photographs of Ladder to the Moon projects on pages 22, 23, 170-175.

Rosemary Lodge Care Home with Nursing (Wimbledon Guild), London.
Thanks to all residents, relatives and staff for the photographs on pages 25, 61, and 112.

David Mitchell for the photo of John Killick and friend on page 96.

Sandra van den Berg for the photographs on pages 14, 80, 81, and 146.

Betty van Gelder for the photograph of her mother on page 41.

Staff photographer for Care Centre St. Jansgeleen, the Netherlands, page 74.

Rende Zoutewelle for the photographs on pages 9, 108, and 167.

Other artwork:

Candy Canzoneri for the drawings on page 154.

Thank you Tineke Poppinga and family for permission to use Jan Poppinga's drawings on pages 76 and 148.

Keri Smith for permission to use the photo of her collage, 'Found city' on page 161.

Every reasonable attempt has been made to identify owners of copyright. Errors or omissions will be corrected in subsequent editions.

ACKNOWLEDGEMENTS

Thank you to Richard Hawkins at Hawker Publications
who was willing to risk on several fronts, and recognised the
soul of this book even before I did; and to Sue Benson for
believing in this book and helping to get it published.
And for her editing, invaluable help with the images,
and support with the book throughout.

Candy Canzoneri, professor of creative writing, was my
reader and cheerleader through this process. Your faith in the
book and in me as the best person to do it, as well as your
humour and insight have been incredibly sustaining.
Thanks for the *creativity disclaimer,* too!

Without the daily online prodding from a group of close
women friends, this book might never have moved out of the
idea stage into the solid object you are holding now. Thank you
Amanda, Carly, Karin, Kathy, Kay Lynne, and Sandy for your
belief in me and your love and encouragement.
And for the bouquet.

Betty van Gelder for your friendship and expert advice on
the typography and help in preparing the book for printing.

Thank you Aunt Evelyn for being such a loyal believer in
my work. Your lively interest, creativity and presence
have softened the loss of my mother (your sister) who
was my number one fan.

Writers usually thank whatever institution gave them the grant
to enable them to work on their book. Mine came from the
'HWH* Foundation'. Without Rende I might not have had the
luxury, after having written the book, to then spend a whole
year to illustrate and design it. Thank you too, for your laughter, support and technical help on all levels, preparing all the
photos, your lovely photographs, and for your steadfastness
during all the ups and downs of this creative process.

*Hard-Working Husbands

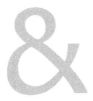

John Killick, Teun
Hamer, Henk Havinga,
Nannie Bos, Monica Blom
and other professional
friends in the field who
valued what I was doing
from the start.

Ed Fisher, Jr. my mentor
and typography teacher
at Carnegie-Mellon
University.

AWgrads, especially
Karen R, Michael N, and
Sandi for your practical
help and friendship.
And Miriam for the
rubber band book.

Brother Hugo, and
Christianne P for
local support.

All my friends, family,
and Rende's family.

Gré
In memoriam

At the nursing home where I worked, there was a lovely lady
who constantly inspired me with her creativity,
warmth, humour and courage.
Every idea I came up with she attempted wholeheartedly.
The doll Samy is hers, her words and spirit
permeate every page of this book.

✝ 2010

ABOUT THE AUTHOR . . . .

Sarah Zoutewelle-Morris was an American artist living in Holland with her fine woodworker husband and their dog Lucie.

She applied her creativity across a wide range of disciplines including graphic design, book design and illustration, calligraphy, fine-art, decoration of period instruments, and working as an artist in health care.

In her creativity workshops and trainings she encouraged people with little or no experience in art to think more creatively and express themselves in a variety of media.

She has written articles on the creative process for the *Journal of Dementia Care* and other publications.

101 Ideas for a Creative Approach to Activities in Dementia Care was her first book. She is also the author of *A Generous Spirit: Exploring New Directions for the Art*

Her web site is: artcalling.wordpress.com

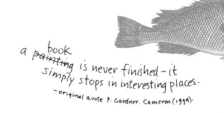

a ~~painting~~ book is never finished – it
simply stops in interesting places.
– original quote P. Gardner. Cameron (1994).

Discover how art can heal, inspire, and bring solace and more meaning to your life

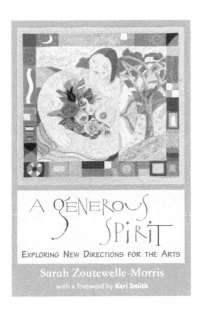

As a trained calligrapher, artist and designer, Sarah Zoutewelle-Morris started out building her career on the 'art as a product' route. Gradually, she came to realize that art is not just products or a vocation, but that it is also intimately connected with healing, transformation and community-building. The process of deep and far-reaching change in herself was influenced by artists she was inspired by.

Art, like friendship, has an intrinsic worth without having to be a means to an end like fame or money. Viewing art as a link to the natural, wild and sacred realms, Sarah's work shifted to seeing art in relationship to others, the world, and generosity.

Sarah contends that it isn't the task of the artist to fit into the market ideology, but rather to bring artistic values, beauty, soaring imagination and fearless skill into that arena. This beautifully illustrated book maps how the arts are a powerful force and how artists are stepping outside the boundaries of the studio, untethered by the emphasis on money, to re-awaken their original function as the intermediary between sacred realms and the newly emerging everyday world. Art is once again fulfilling its visionary role in creation and renewal, offering fresh images to light up our imagination and alternatives to how to live on our planet. Art can transform you: it can awaken your generous spirit.

186 pages
ISBN 978-1-912698-98-1 (paperback)
ISBN 978-1-912698-99-8 (ebook)
Published by Kaminn Media
kaminnmedia.com

Lightning Source UK Ltd.
Milton Keynes UK
UKHW020927091221
395320UK00003B/54